L A S E R S

IN ORTHOPAEDICS

L A S E R S

IN ORTHOPAEDICS

Edited by

Henry H. Sherk, M.D.

Professor of Surgery
Chief, Division of Orthopaedics and Rehabilitation
The Medical College of Pennsylvania
Philadelphia, Pennsylvania

J. B. LIPPINCOTT COMPANY
Philadelphia

Grand Rapids • New York • St. Louis • San Francisco
London • Sydney • Tokyo

Acquisitions Editor: *Darlene Barela Cooke*
Developmental Editor: *Delois Patterson*
Project Editor: *Melissa B. McElroy*
Copy Editor: *Diane Lamsback*
Indexer: *Ellen Murray*
Designer: *Doug Smock*
Design Coordinator: *Doug Smock*
Production Manager: *Carol A. Florence*
Production Coordinator: *Kathryn Rule*
Compositor: *Digitype*
Printer/Binder: *R.R. Donnelley & Sons*

1   3   5   6   4   2

Library of Congress Cataloging in Publication Data

Lasers in Orthopaedics.
    Includes index.
    1. Orthopedic surgery.   2. Lasers in surgery.
I. Sherk, Henry H., 1930–   . [DNLM: 1. Laser
Surgery.   2. Orthopedics.   WE 168 L343]
RD732.L37   1990   617.3   89-12347
ISBN 0-397-50962-6

The authors and publisher have exerted every effort to ensure that drug
selection and dosage set forth in this text are in accord with current recommendations and practice at the time of publication. However, in view of
ongoing research, changes in government regulations, and the constant flow
of information relating to drug therapy and drug reactions, the reader is
urged to check the package insert for each drug for any change in indications and dosage and for added warnings and precautions. This is particularly important when the recommended agent is a new or infrequently
employed drug.

To my wife, Lea

Contributors

Steven P. Arnoczky, D.V.M., DPL A.C.V.S.
Laboratory of Comparative
  Orthopaedics
The Hospital for Special Surgery
New York, New York

John D. Cunningham, M.D.
Surgical Research Fellow
Department of Surgery and the
  Reichle Surgical Research
  Laboratory
Temple University
Philadelphia, Pennsylvania

Stephen V. Fealy
New York, New York

W. Edward Johansen, M.D.
Los Angeles, California

Anne M. Kelly, B.A.
Medical Student
The State University of New
  York, Buffalo
Buffalo, New York

Charles Kollmer, M.D.
Clinical Instructor in
  Orthopaedics
Medical College of Pennsylvania
Philadelphia, Pennsylvania
Attending Physician
North Penn Hospital
Lansdale, Pennsylvania

G. June Marshall, Ph.D.
Orthopaedic Hospital Medical
  Center
Los Angeles, California

Menachem M. Meller, M.D., Ph.D.
Assistant Instructor
Division of Orthopaedics and
  Rehabilitation
The Medical College of
  Pennsylvania
Philadelphia, Pennsylvania

Drew V. Miller, M.D.
Chief Orthopaedic Resident
The Hospital for Special Surgery
New York, New York

Stephen J. O'Brien, M.D.
The Hospital for Special Surgery
Assistant Attending
  Orthopaedic Surgeon
The New York Hospital
Assistant Professor of Surgery
Cornell University Medical
  School
Chief Orthopaedic Consultant
St. John's University
Assistant Team Physician
New York Giants Football
New York, New York

Anthony L. B. Rhodes, M.D.
Medical College of Pennsylvania
Philadelphia, Pennsylvania

Joaquin Sariego, M.D.
Medical College of Pennsylvania
Philadelphia Veterans
  Administration Hospital
Rolling Hill Hospital
Philadelphia, Pennsylvania

Bernard Sigel, M.D.
Professor and Chairman
The Department of Surgery
The Medical College of
  Pennsylvania
Philadelphia, Pennsylvania

Chadwick F. Smith, M.D.
Clinical Professor of
  Orthopaedic Surgery
University of Southern
  California
Los Angeles, California

Richard Smith, M.D.
Medical College of Pennsylvania
Philadelphia, Pennsylvania

Leroy V. Sutter, Jr., Ph.D.
Directed Energy, Inc.
Los Angeles, California

Gurvinder S. Uppal, M.D.
Assistant Instructor
Division of Orthopaedics and
  Rehabilitation
Medical College of Pennsylvania
Philadelphia, Pennsylvania

C. Thomas Vangsness, M.D.
Orthopaedic Hospital Medical
  Center
LAC/USC Medical Center
Los Angeles, California

Russell F. Warren, M.D.
Director of Sports Medicine
The Hospital for Special Surgery
Professor of Orthopaedics
Cornell University Medical
  Center
Attending Physician
The New York Hospital
New York, New York

John V. White, M.D., F.A.C.S.
Associate Professor of Surgery
Director of Surgical Research
Temple University Hospital
Philadelphia, Pennsylvania

**Howard A. Zaren, M.D.,
  F.A.C.S.**
Professor of Surgery
Chief, Division of General
  Surgery
Vice-Chairman, Department of
  Surgery
Medical College of Pennsylvania
Philadelphia, Pennsylvania

Preface

The acquisition of the first laser by virtually any hospital is probably a nonevent for the orthopaedic staff at that institution. This was certainly the case at the hospital of the Medical College of Pennsylvania several years ago, when surgeons in other disciplines began to operate with the CO_2 lasers initially purchased by M.C.P. During the ensuing months, as the general surgeons and others gradually developed greater interest and skill in the use of these devices, orthopaedists realized that we were nonparticipants in an apparently exciting new technology. Partly from this sense of being left out, we began to seek possible uses for lasers in musculoskeletal surgery. A literature search revealed only a few published papers on laser applications in orthopaedics, but these offered glimpses into a whole new realm of possibilities. Laser arthroscopy, laser revision arthroplasty, tissue welding, tumor therapy with lasers, laser discectomy, and even controlling cellular metabolism with lasers suddenly seemed like potential realities.

Despite our curiosity and desire to begin laser surgery, it was not possible for orthopaedic surgeons merely to begin to apply the laser to our practices. The use of these devices is governed by hospital regulations that require surgeons to document training in laser surgery in their respective specialties. We experienced considerable difficulty in handling this. The lack of an organized body of information concerning lasers in orthopaedic surgery and the impossibility of finding a course to attend made us realize the necessity for a text that would address these needs. It is our hope that this book will correct the deficiencies we encountered and we offer it in the expectation that it will help other orthopaedists learn about and better understand lasers. We also hope that by identifying and bringing together the core of knowledge concerning lasers in orthopaedics, certifying bodies such as hospital laser safety committees will understand that lasers do have a role in musculoskeletal surgery. We think the book should, for this reason, help orthopaedic surgeons become certified more readily to use lasers in their practices.

Two years ago, I was privileged to present a paper on "What's New in Orthopaedics" at the meeting of the American College of Surgeons. I realized while preparing for this, that although orthopaedic surgery is a growing field with an expanding knowledge base, there does seem to be a sameness to the papers and discussions on, for example, total joint replacement, fracture fixation, and spine surgery. Much of what one reads and reviews about orthopaedic surgery are refinements and very gradual advances in familiar subjects. The concept of lasers in orthopaedics, however, is truly new. The possibilities are dramatic and exciting and it appears that lasers may open new vistas for orthopaedists. We, as musculoskeletal surgeons, have little or no background in the technology of lasers and certainly no collective experience. It will take time, patience, and honest, unbiased reporting to establish the place of lasers in surgery of the musculoskeletal system; therefore, this book is offered as a first statement in what may become an important technology in our field. The advances in laser science are occurring so rapidly that the laser in use today, may well be outmoded tomorrow. Nevertheless, there has to be a starting point, and this book is written in the hope and expectation that surgeons in future years will build upon it.

In this spirit, the author is indebted to a number of individuals. The orthopaedic resident staff at the Medical College of Pennsylvania, in particular, has devoted its energy, talent, and enthusiasm to the basic research and clinical applications of lasers in orthopaedics. This small group (Dr. John Nolan, Dr. Charles Kollmer, Dr. Richard Smith, Dr. Gurvinder Uppal, Dr. Menachem Meller, and Dr. Anthony Rhodes) with its very large clinical responsibilities has been able to sustain its effort and interest in this new field and has made a very real contribution. I am also indebted to my colleagues, Dr. James Bassett, former chairman of the Department of Surgery at the Medical College of Pennsylvania, Dr. Bernard Sigel, current chairman at MCP, and especially Dr. Howard Zaren, chief of General Surgery.

Dr. Zaren's interest in our use of lasers in orthopaedics and continued support have been essential to our work and have been a major stimulus. I am also indebted to Dr. Chadwick Smith of the University of Southern California and Dr. Stephen O'Brien of the Hospital for Special Surgery in New York, for permitting me to visit them and observe their laser techniques in arthroscopic surgery. Dr. John White of Temple University in Philadelphia is one of the pioneers in the use of lasers in tissue welding and has shared his knowledge and experience with us on many occasions. I am grateful to him for this and for his contributions to this text. I must also mention Mr. Alden Ludlow and Mr. Ted Belleza of Heraus Lasersonics and Mr. Robert Hoffman of Sharplan Lasers, who have helped with their input and assistance. My friend, Mr. Joseph T. Rothrock, IV, medical photographer extraordinaire, also has made a major contribution, not only with excellent intraoperative photography, but also with counsel and advice. Thanks are also due to Dr. John Gartland, who read portions of this manuscript and helped me organize my thoughts. Finally I must acknowledge my gratitude to my wife, Lea, who after 25 years still does not object to the time it takes to do this kind of thing. This book is affectionately dedicated to her.

Henry H. Sherk, M.D.

Contents

Arthroscopic Surgery with a Contact Nd:YAG Laser   158

Anne M. Kelly, Stephen J. O'Brien, Drew V. Miller, Stephen V. Fealy, and Russell F. Warren

Arthroscopic Surgery with the CO$_2$ Laser Wave Guide   168
Henry H. Sherk, Menachem M. Meller, and Anthony Rhodes

1

Introduction
to Lasers

Menachem M. Meller

A laser (light amplification by stimulated emission of radiation) is a device that produces electromagnetic energy. It requires three essential elements: a lasing medium, a means of reflecting electromagnetic energy back into the medium, and an energy source (Fig. 1–1). The atoms or molecules of the lasing medium are contained in a chamber initially in an unenergized or ground state. Upon absorbing mechanical, thermal, or optical energy, these atoms or molecules are raised to a higher electronic or kinetic energy state by outward displacement of electrons from inner valence rings. If the molecule releases the energy as electromagnetic radiation, a process of spontaneous emission occurs with release of packets or quanta of energy. This process occurs in the production of light in a neon sign, for example. In a laser, however, the quanta are reflected back into already energized molecules by reflective surfaces at the ends of the chamber. A second generation of quanta is then released that is identical to the first in wavelength and direction. Because one of the reflective surfaces is made partially transparent, the light amplified by the stimulated emission of radiation can escape from one end of the chamber as a laser beam.

The beam of the laser is unlike an ordinary thermal light source in that it is columnated, coherent, and monochromatic (Fig. 1-2). Collimated means that the rays in the beam do not diverge over distance. *Monochromicity* means that within narrow limits, each ray in the beam has the same wavelength. *Coherence* means that the wavelength is stable both spatially and temporally.

From a surgical standpoint, collimation assures complete delivery of the laser beam as well as focusing ability. Monochromicity is

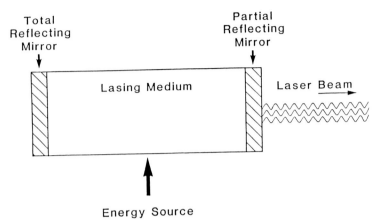

Figure 1–1. Schematic diagram illustrating the three essential components of a laser device: lasing medium, lasing chamber, and energy source.

useful when one tissue will selectively take up the given laser beam. Coherence is not generally a useful property for surgery.

The specific change in the tissue depends on the quanta absorbed. A quanta of ultraviolet light alters the state of excitation of the outer electronic structure of the molecules, those involved in ionization and chemical reaction. A quantum of visible or near infrared energy will alter the state of molecular vibration. Microwave energy will alter the state of molecular rotation. X-rays alter the energy of the

Figure 1–2. Illustration of the difference between the electromagnetic energy emanating from a thermal light source such as an incandescent light bulb versus a laser light. In a laser, the rays in the beam are columnated (travel in parallel lines), monochromatic (the height and spacing of the peaks and valleys are identical), and coherent (the peaks and valleys line up).

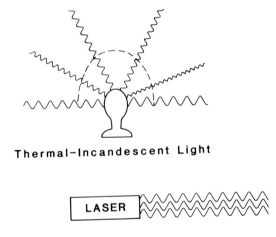

inner nonvalent electrons. In absolute terms, a photon in the near infrared range contains one electron volt. In the ultraviolet range, it contains 100 electron volts. In the x-ray range, it contains 10,000 electron volts. Ultimately, visible and near infrared radiation can only cause heating effects in the tissue (*i.e.*, coagulation and vaporization) (Fig. 1–3).

Lasers are identified by their lasing medium. Until recently, four lasers were in common use in medicine—carbon dioxide (CO_2), neodymium: yttrium aluminum garnet (Nd:YAG), argon, and krypton. Selection of a given laser is based on its wavelength, its power capability, and the means of delivering this laser beam through the tissue (Table 1–1).

In a CO_2 laser, the lasing medium is actually filled with a mixture of CO_2, nitrogen, and helium gas. It emits energy at 10.6 μ in the infrared range of the electromagnetic spectrum. It is highly efficient at converting the input energy into laser energy, allowing high-power output. Its depth of penetration at any instant in time is limited by the water content in the tissues to about 50 μ. There is

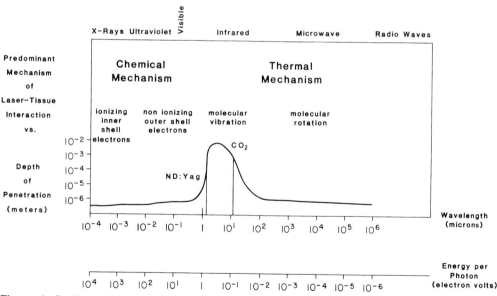

Figure 1–3. The electromagnetic spectrum. The effects of the commonly used surgical lasers on tissue are thermal and are affected by increases in rotation and vibration of the constituent molecules. The depth of penetration into tissue varies with the specific wavelength of the laser being used. The energy per photon as a function of wavelength is shown on the lower scale.

3

Table 1–1
Operating Characteristics of Surgical Lasers

Laser Type	Maximum Power (watts)	Major Wavelength (μm)	Depth of Penetration (μm)	Delivery System
CO_2	0–100	10.6	50	Articulated arm, semi-rigid and fiberoptic
Nd:YAG	0–100	1.6	10,000	Fiberoptic cable
Argon	0–20	0.49	300	Fiberoptic cable
		0.51		
Krypton	0–10	550–598 nm	200	Fiberoptic cable
Excimer (xenon cloride) experimental	0–100	308 nm	100	Fiberoptic cable

little scattering of the laser in the neighboring tissues. This laser is good for cutting, but not coagulating. It is useful for incisions in soft tissues and cartilage, where a good depth and width control are needed. It is less useful for bone with little water content, or for removing large volumes of tissue.

In a Nd:YAG laser, the lasing medium is a solid crystal of yitrium aluminum garnet doped with about 3% neodymium. The crystal matrix alters the electron configuration of the neodymium, making stimulated emissions possible. The output wavelength is 1.064 μ in the near infrared range of the electromagnetic spectrum. This laser, too, is one with high output of about 100 watts. Its depth of penetration into tissue at any given instant in time is about 1 cm or 1600 times that of a CO_2 laser. There is much scattering into the neighboring tissue, making this laser useful for coagulation, but not for cutting. To cut or evaporate a volume of tissue equivalent to that cut or evaporated by a CO_2 laser would require 500 times the power output. Water does not absorb the beam of the Nd:YAG laser; therefore, this laser can be used on wet tissues or endoscopically. Blood and other pigments strongly absorb the rays, causing local heating with tissue damage and preventing further penetration.

Argon and krypton lasers are both visible light-range lasers, about 0.48 μ, 0.51 μ, and 0.55–0.60 μ respectively. Both lasers are low power (about 1 watt) and have excellent depth penetration, but highly variable absorptive scattering and reflective properties. Pigmented tissues strongly absorb the beam, nonhomogeneous nonpigmented tissues scatter it, and clear, watery tissues transmit it. These lasers are used primarily in ophthalmology for retinal photocoagulation and in dermatology for removal of pigmented dermal lesions.

Throughout this book, we will provide basic information on how to select a laser for a given clinical task. Whenever possible, specific clinical applications will be stressed. Orthopaedics has been lagging behind some of the other surgical specialties in employing the laser. This may soon change, however, especially as newer eximer lasers operating in the ultraviolet range become available. These hold the promise of being able to cut through dense bone and cartilage by a cool, chemolytic method.

2

Laser Delivery Systems

Charles Kollmer

The numbers and types of lasers in use are expanding rapidly. Several commonly used medical lasers are available in most hospitals. An understanding of what kinds of lasers are available and their potential uses is required. The power range, adaptability, wavelength, protective measures, operative set-up, and tissue effects are all germaine to proper utilization of these machines. Several commonly used medical lasers are described in Table 2–1. Description of the various laser features is presented along with a listing of the various lasers with essential parameters. New lasers and new uses for these lasers are constantly emerging.

Because of the laser's range of power, the output can be varied to the optimal level (power density) to perform the needed function.

Variation of power input, mode, or focus can be used to affect laser power output. The intensity of the laser beam can be modified by manipulation of the gating mechanism, which produces the following different laser modes:

1. Continuous wave. Direct constant opening of the gate for the duration of the laser use.
2. Pulse (gated). Intermittent stoppage of the continuous wave for short time intervals (*e.g.*, 0.1 sec/sec). This is not the same as a true pulsed laser, but this is what is commonly referred to in the medical community as a "pulsed laser." The result is a cooler laser beam with energy levels equivalent to those achieved with the continuous beam.
3. Superpulse. The storing up of laser power in the optical cavity of the laser and the use of a very fast shutter to release

(text continued on page 10)

Table 2–1
Medical Lasers

Type	Wavelength	Power Range	Modes	Response and Uses
Far Infrared Spectrum				
CO_2	10,600 nm	0–100 watts	C,P,SP	High water absorption
Mid-Infrared Spectrum				
Erb:YAG	2900 nm	—	—	Very high water absorption
Hydrogen fluoride	2500 nm	0–3 watts	C,P	Cutting/moderate coagulation
Holmium	2100 nm	—	—	
Near Infrared Spectrum				
Nd:YAG	1064–1320 nm	0–125 watts	C,P,SP	High protein absorption
Gallium–arsenide	830–904 nm	—	C,P	—
Dysprosium	—	—	—	—
Visible Spectrum				
KTP	532 nm	0–15 watts	P	Pigment (red, black) absorption
Argon	488–515 nm	0–15 watts	C,P,SP	Pigment (red, black) absorption

	Wavelength	Power	Mode	Use
Krypton	598–612 nm	—	C,P	Pigment (red, black) absorption
Copper	578 nm	0–15 watts	P	Pigment (red, black) absorption
Gold	630 nm	0–15 watts	P	Pigment (red, black) absorption
Dye (tunable, solid-state, argon-pumped)				
Red	630 nm	0–10 watts	C,P	Photosensitized-tumor irradiation
Yellow	577 nm	0–10 watts	C,P	Vascular-tissue ablation
Green	504 nm	0–10 watts	C,P	Pigment (red, black) absorption
Helium–neon	630 nm	0–50 milliwatts	C	Ideal aiming beam with "cold" lase
Ruby	630 nm	1–3 watts	C,P	Ophthalmic surgery
Ultraviolet Spectrum				
Excimer				
Krypton–fluoride	308 nm	Milliwatts	C,P	Photoablation
Xenon–chloride	248 nm	Milliwatts	C,P	Usable for hard tissue
Argon–fluoride	193 nm	Milliwatts	C,P	Usable for hard tissue
Free-electron	Theoretically unlimited wavelength and power range			Experimental

P, pulse; C, continuous; SP, superpulse.

short-duration, high-intensity laser bursts. This is a combination of pulsing and continuous-wave application, and the energy is measured in an integral fashion (*e.g.*, 35-watt superpulse = sufficient number of 500-watt bursts averaged over a 1-sec interval). The effect is strong cutting power with less heat build-up.

4. Pulse (true). Intermittent and high build-up of energy within the optical cavity. The energy released is of short duration on the order of microseconds or less. The power generated is higher than can be achieved with the continuous beam. The pulses are of short duration, and emitted energy is measured in milliwatts. These lasers are not useful for orthopedic applications at this time.

5. Q-Switching (giant pulse). Extremely high energy production on the order of millions of watts for extremely short periods of time (nano-, pico-, or femtoseconds). This effect is achieved within special dye cells or by an electro-optic "cell" within the resonator. Mode locking, a similar process, will produce series of these bursts. The effect is nonthermal (nonlinear) photodisruption of incident tissue. These effects are of great interest for the possibility of nonthermal surgical application to orthopaedic tissues, although this is still experimental.

The diameter of the laser beam also impacts on its power. The power density (watt per square centimeter) refers to laser power in terms of surface area of "spot size", therefore, the small spot size will have a greater power density for any particular power rating. With a CO_2 laser, for example,

10 watts of power at 0.2-mm spot size =
28.0 kilowatts of power density

10 watts of power at 1.0-mm spot size =
3.1 kilowatts of power density

The power density in this case is a matter of focal length, which, in turn, determines the spot size. By changing the focal length, spot size and, therefore, power density, can be varied.

Directly increasing or decreasing the input from the high-voltage pump source also allows one to manipulate power density.

CO$_2$ LASERS

This laser is the most frequently used medical laser. This laser emits radiation in the far infrared range and is highly absorbed by water. The lasing medium is a mixture of CO$_2$, nitrogen, and helium. Because the CO$_2$ laser beam is invisible, an aiming beam laser is also needed. Usually a nonthermal helium-neon laser is used for aiming purposes. The gaseous mixture is usually replenished by means of tanks in most large hospital-based systems. The power range for these devices is substantial, it ranges from the milliwatt level to over 100 watts. Smaller, closed CO$_2$ systems are also available. These smaller lasers are radio-frequency controlled. The radio-frequency signal acts upon the lasing medium to produce a beam with power ranges that are narrower than those seen with the open systems. The advantages of portability, constant closed supply, and low voltage requirements make these smaller lasers attractive for office-based uses. The power ranges are narrower up to approximately 20 watts.

Because of the high water absorption, the CO$_2$ laser is a good cutting instrument that has some coagulation effects (0.1 mm). Also, CO$_2$-laser energy is highly absorbed by quartz, silicone, and other fiberoptic materials. This renders it unusable with standard fiberoptic cables. New waveguides have been recently developed for guiding CO$_2$ lasers in difficult access areas. Limitations in length and flexibility are noteworthy. The length of most waveguides cannot exceed approximately 45 cm, and these devices are able to bend usually no more than 30 degrees. The waveguides are discussed in more detail with laser delivery systems. The standard for CO$_2$ lasers is the focusing handpiece or microscope.

Nd:YAG LASERS

The Nd:YAG is another workhorse laser. The beam is produced by means of flashlamp excitation of the neodymium (Nd)-impregnated YAG (yttrium aluminum garnet) crystal. The laser beam produced is fiberoptic capable and has a wide power range (0 watts – 100 watts). The Nd:YAG laser is highly absorbed by protein and evidences a significant coagulation zone of 4 mm to 6 mm. This coagulation effect is very large, particularly in comparison with the 0.1-mm coagulation zones noted with the CO$_2$ laser. Thin fibers down to approximately 250 μ can be used for multiple endoscopic procedures. Also, the thermal effects can be minimized with Q-switching. This capability can be used to advantage for lithotripsy (removal of renal or biliary stones).

Another aspect of the Nd:YAG laser is the use of contact tips. Sapphire contact tips of various shapes have been utilized to decrease the coagulating effect and maximize the cutting capabilities with the Nd:YAG laser. The use of hollow contact tips is also a possibility. Theoretically, one gets a combination of the purely thermal effect from the tip and the radiation effect particular to the wavelength of the laser's beam. The contact tips require direct application; otherwise, the tip may burn up. The return of tactile sensation with this device is also advantageous.

ARGON LASERS

The Argon laser produces light in the blue 488-nm range and the green 515-nm range. High absorption by red and black pigments is responsible for the utility of this fiberoptic-capable laser on vascular tissue. This laser has a power range of 0 watts to 15 watts and requires high energy input as well as fiber cooling. It is adaptable for microscope control and also may be outfitted with contact tips. The contact tips are composed of metal and provide purely thermal effects. Hollow tips have also been used with the argon laser for removal of atheromatous plaques.

The coagulation effect of the noncontact argon laser falls between that of the CO_2 and Nd:YAG lasers at approximately 1.0 mm. This would make the argon laser a good instrument for most dissection except for its narrow power range and high energy requirements.

KTP LASERS

The potassium titanyl phosphate (KTP) laser is produced by means of frequency doubling the output from a Nd:YAG laser by means of an electro-optical crystal. This effect produces a light beam of pure 532-nm wavelength. The green light of the KTP laser recognizes red and black pigments well. The laser is adaptable to any mode and is used with microscope, handpiece, and fiberoptic systems. The beam is pulsed and requires no fiber cooling, which is advantageous in closed spaces (*e.g.*, the peritoneal cavity). The power range for the KTP laser is the same as that for the argon laser.

DYE LASERS

Tunable dye lasers are produced by excitation of jets of various colored dyes. The energy source is usually an argon laser or flash-lamps. The tunability comes from changing the dye or modulating the electro-optics; it is not just a matter of changing a dial. The turnover of the dye laser to a different wavelength requires a good bit of time and labor. The colors that can be obtained are very pure. The red lasers are used for irradiation of photosensitized tumors because of their superior depth of penetration into the tissue. The yellow lasers are used for ablation of vascular tissue because of their excellent absorption by hemoglobin and pulse characteristics that minimize thermal conduction to surrounding tissue. The green lasers are used for endoscopic purposes, including lithotripsy, and also in recanalization of vessels.

KRYPTON AND RUBY LASERS

Krypton and ruby lasers are used almost exclusively in ophthalmic surgery. The power ranges and wavelengths are apparently not of value for use in the musculoskeletal tissues.

HELIUM – NEON LASERS

The helium–neon laser has multiple uses. Its beam is visible and bright, making it an ideal aiming beam. The production of the helium–neon laser is cost effective, and the laser is easily adapted to coaxial purpose. The laser is used in the 10-milliwatt to 50-milliwatt range and as such provides minimal to no thermal effect on the incident tissue. The use of the helium–neon laser for bioregulatory effects is presented in a separate chapter.

EXCIMER LASERS

The excimer (excited dimer) lasers are very attractive for use in orthopaedics. These ultraviolet lasers can be used for nonthermal photodisruption effects with high power ranges. A precise laser osteotomy with absolute minimal thermal necrosis was recently reported for in vitro trials on cortical bone. Fiberoptic capability also makes arthroscopic use a possibility.

Work is ongoing to produce a tunable laser crystal that can be easily modulated over a very wide range from infrared to ultraviolet. This laser will not be available for several years, but early tests have been successful.

FREE-ELECTRON LASERS

It will take years for the free-electron laser to be perfected and ready for application in the medical fields. The idea of a laser without any particular lasing medium is very attractive, but the expense and size of present units are still prohibitive.

OTHER LASERS

Research with the lasers discussed in the preceding sections is continuing. The effect of each laser are dependent on power and wavelength. Mid-infrared lasers show very high specificity for water and thus are good for cutting with minimal coagulation effects. The erbium (Erb):YAG laser can be used for osteotomies with minimal thermal necrosis. The research for this type of effect is preliminary and undergoing bench research trials at this time. The erbium:YAG, gallium–arsenide, holmium, and dysprosium lasers have all been investigated for clinical use as "soft" lasers.

CURRENT DELIVERY SYSTEMS

As described earlier, production of the laser beam occurs in the resonating chamber. The efficiency of beam production is variable, depending on the substrate. Heat is generated in the resonating chamber as a result of this energy loss, so an effective means of cooling is required. Both gas (nitrogen, CO_2, and air, etc.) and water-cooled systems are available. Some units use recirculating coolant to allow greater portability.

In gas-substrate lasers (*e.g.*, CO_2), constant replenishment of the medium is important to keep the gas mixtures balanced and also to avoid by-product build-up at the electrodes. This can be managed with an open or closed self-contained system. The advantages of portability are gained at the expense of overall efficiency and power range. Most office-type, low-wattage lasers utilize closed systems. Waste gas is removed from the resonator and either is flushed out of the system or recirculated. Major in-hospital lasers usually involve open gas systems in which regular tank changes are required.

FIBEROPTICS

Once the laser beam is generated, it is necessary to conduct the beam to the target. The use of fiberoptics lends itself well to this, and most available lasers are fiberoptic capable, except for the CO_2 laser (10,600 nm), which is not transmittable through fibers. The CO_2 laser heats the fiber and destroys it.

A cross-sectional diagram shows the components found in a fiberoptic cable (Fig. 2–1). The inner transmitting fiber is usually a thin, brittle, translucent material such as silica, quartz, glass, or other compound. This inner fiber is the regulating factor for beam transmission. The commonly used fibers have a wide range of transmissible wavelengths from ultraviolet to near infrared, and the spe-

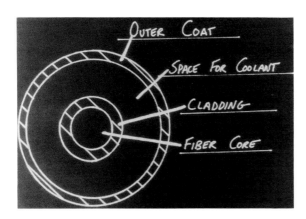

Figure 2–1. Diagrammatic cross section of fiberoptic cable.

15

cifics of each fiber should be matched for the wavelength characteristics of each laser. The fibers used with lasers are single-core cables, and, depending upon fiber length and absorption characteristics, there is a relative power loss in the transmission process. Immediately adjacent to the core is the cladding. The cladding is composed of a flexible substance (silicon, teflon, or urethane-type materials). The bending characteristics of these materials keep the brittle inner core intact (Fig. 2–2). The next layer is the outer lining, or coat, which is usually composed of a very bendable material. Between the cladding and the outer coat, a thin space is often left to allow coolant (gas or fluid) to be forced along the entire fiber. The coolant is particularly important at the tip, where the laser is emitted. Here, small imperfections in the fiber tip will cause absorption of a portion of the laser energy. Should this occur, the fiber tip could rapidly heat up and be destroyed.

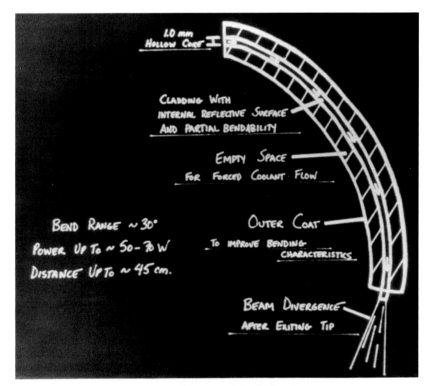

Figure 2–2. Diagrammatic longitudinal section of laser fiberoptic cable.

The end of the fiber usually has an adapter to keep all parts of the cable together. These fibers are meant for noncontact use. Applying the tip directly on tissue will cause a rapid build-up in temperature and damage the tip. If a smooth tip surface is not maintained, heating of the tip and misaiming of the beam occurs. Repair of fiber tips is part of the laser staff's duty. Spare fibers should always be available and in good condition to avoid delay or mishap in the middle of a procedure. Commercially produced disposable fibers are also available.

Control of the laser spot size is also an important consideration with the fibers. The beam is not focused using a conventional lens system. The beam diverges continuously from exit at the fiber tip (Fig. 2–3), and the power density at the tip is the highest. The surgeon controls the proximity to the target; thus, the effective power density on the tissue is controlled. As already noted, the tips are not meant for tissue contact.

Various contact tips have been designed and used for clinical purposes. Metal tips for heat conduction have been used successfully in angioplasty systems. Tips of various shapes and with different functional capabilities are also available. The sapphire contact tip has probably received the most attention, particularly when used with the Nd:YAG laser. A combination form of contact tip is hollow

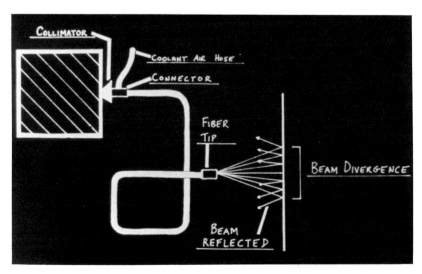

Figure 2–3. Diagram of fiberoptic cable showing collimator, coolant, and fiber tip. There is divergence of the beam from the tip of the fiber.

in the center. This configuration can be used to maximize the ablative characteristics of the thermal contact tip and the coagulative aspects of the particular laser used. By using a contact tip, the surgeon regains the advantage of tactile response.

Fibers used for image transmission require multiple fibers, sometimes thousands of fibers, but the fibers used for surgical laser transmission use single-fiber cores and thus are not useful for imaging.

ARMATURES

The CO_2 laser has a long wavelength in the far infrared zone (10,600 nm) that is really absorbed by the fiberoptic core; this results in poor transmission, severe power loss, and rapid destruction of the fiberoptic cable. This is a problem, because the CO_2 laser is the most commonly used surgical laser. The delivery system for the CO_2 laser is a series of mirrored armatures (Fig. 2–4). The reflective surfaces within the armature are composed of various substances (*e.g.*, germanium). The collimated beam maintains its power with this system. The laser beam is then focused at the handpiece to bring it to a reasonable spot size for surgical use. The power density varies with spot size, and the spot size is determined by the focusing system and the distance from the target tissue. By changing the focal length of

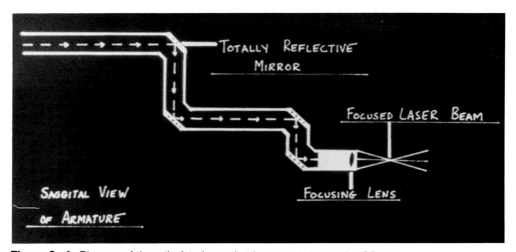

Figure 2–4. Diagram of the articulated arm that is currently in use for CO_2 lasers.

the lens, handpieces of different sizes can be used. Most systems work in the 50-mm to 250-mm range.

Alignment of the mirrors is important for proper aiming and power. Alignment is checked prior to use of the laser by assuring that the CO_2 laser is aimed at the same spot as the aiming beam. The aiming beam is usually a low-level helium–neon laser. This procedure should be repeated every time the laser is used. Also, if the surgeon notes a decreased effectiveness or that the handpiece becomes hot while using the CO_2 laser, the proper alignment of the beam should be checked.

With available systems, the body of the laser can be kept several feet away from the operative field. The use of balanced armatures and multiple "knuckles" gives as much freedom as possible with this less-than-fiberoptic method.

MICROSCOPE

Using the same principle of beam focusing with an optical lens, a microscope can be adapted to deliver the beam to the target tissue. The size of the beam can be extremely small (0.1 mm–0.2 mm or less). This device keeps the surgical field clear of instrumentation and increases operator control. Focusing of the beam to 300 mm or more is possible. A micromanipulator, or "joystick," can be employed to provide precision aiming. Coupling with a variable focus–defocus device increases the utility of the microscope. The microscope also can be coupled with a computer to create precise laser patterns.

WAVEGUIDE

Fiberoptic systems obviously have great advantage for percutaneous, endoscopic, and laparoscopic use. The utility for arthroscopy is evident. The characteristics of each laser must be taken into account when providing the delivery system and operating environment. The Nd:YAG laser is fiberoptic capable in a fluid or gaseous medium, but the CO_2 laser requires a gaseous medium. Several investigators have used armature-based CO_2 lasers for arthroscopy with varying results. There has been a long search for a good CO_2 fiberoptic system. The newest developments involve waveguide technology. A waveguide has a hollow core that transmits the beam, with some loss of power as distance increases. The cladding in the waveguide is a reflective material (*e.g.,* metals). The result of these designs is a loss of flexibility when compared with fiberoptic cables. Also, owing to the power loss, the waveguides are restricted in length. Several types of waveguide are now available. Most provide 50 watts to 70 watts of continuous wave, with lengths up to approximately 45 cm and bendability to approximately 30 degrees.

The waveguide systems have been used in laparoscopic procedures. The problems of smoke evacuation and maintenance of pneumoperitoneum are similar to the anticipated difficulties one would find in arthroscopy. New evacuation instrumentation developed to deal with laparoscopic use has proved useful.

SMOKE EVACUATORS

Discussion of smoke evacuators seems appropriate at this point. The laser "plume" is a controversial topic, particularly in light of reports suggesting viral inoculation of surgical personnel. Live human papilloma virus (HPV) particles have been retrieved from condyloma excision plumes. This report has been questioned by several investigators. The issue of safety is a concern, and an effective method of smoke evacuation is mandatory. These devices use high-power suction and filtration to purify the smoke. Filtration to approximately $0.12\ \mu$ is available in present commercial evacuators. (It is necessary that the vacuum device be positioned for maximal clearance of the laser plume so that visualization of the surgical field is not impeded.) A separate discussion of the laser plume is presented in Chapter 3 (Laser Safety).

CONCLUSION

Surgical experience with each of the laser delivery systems is important for proper use and understanding of the advantages and limitations of each system. As laser surgery advances, more hardware will be necessary because of the great potential for percutaneous surgery. The combination of laser fiber or waveguide, computer with appropriate software program, television and VCR, and laser feedback and diagnostic equipment is already a possibility in cardio-vascular angioplasty surgery. Certainly, similar applications can be envisioned for orthopaedics. As more surgical applications come into clinical use, the choice of the appropriate laser and availability of the delivery system become an issue.

3

Laser Safety

Henry H. Sherk
Menachem Meller

The surgical use of lasers offers the advantages of noncontact surgery, a dry surgical field, precisely localized tissue ablation, and sterile wounds. Nevertheless, lasers have the potential for harm, not only to the patient but also to the surgeons, nurses, and all other personnel in the operating-room environment. It is the responsibility of all who work in this environment to ensure the safe use of these devices. In the recognition of the need for laser safety, there are a number of agencies that set standards for, authorize, and control the use of lasers. These agencies are the American National Standards Institute (ANSI), Food and Drug Administration (FDA), the AMA Council on Scientific Affairs, state and local regulatory agencies, and local hospital boards and committees that delineate privileges for laser use.

Safety standards for lasers have been detailed in the ANSI volumes Z136 and Z136.1.[1] The standards established by ANSI represent general agreement among manufacturers, sales personnel, and users regarding the best current practices. These standards have been largely adopted by the panel on Lasers in Medicine and Surgery established by the AMA Council on Scientific Affairs.[6] Although the FDA recognizes and utilizes the standards, it does not directly regulate the use of lasers in clinical practice. The FDA, through the Medical Device Amendments under the Food, Drug and Cosmetics Act, is empowered by Congress to regulate the producers of lasers and approve or disapprove the sale of laser devices for specific applications. The National Center for Medical Devices and Radiologic Health has the responsibility of enforcing FDA regulations.[2] The FDA does not prohibit a physician from using a laser in a clinical situation if the physician feels that the laser is the best tool for a specific patient. For data collection and clinical testing of lasers, however, the FDA requires an investigational device exemption (IDE) prior to the use of the laser. In general, therefore, the use of lasers by physicians is locally regulated by hospital governance procedures and requires approval and accreditation by committees supervising appointments and delineation of privileges in the clinical setting. The FDA also regulates lasers through the Radiation Control Act and must certify lasers as free of radiation hazards. Lasers that are currently available for medical uses do not emit ionizing irradiation and so are not subject to this legislation.[11]

CERTIFICATION OF PHYSICIANS FOR USE OF LASERS

In accordance with the standards developed by ANSI and adopted by the AMA Council of Scientific Affairs, most hospitals require documentation of instruction in lasers before allowing a staff physician laser privileges. In order to obtain the necessary documentation, it has usually been necessary for the physicians and surgeons to take an instructional course in lasers. In most circumstances, the available courses provide 5 hours of didactic instruction in laser physics and safety and an additional 5 hours of hands-on experience. It should be noted that instruction is usually required for different types of lasers because of their varying effects on tissues and safety requirements. Thus, instruction in the use of the CO_2 laser is not adequate for the use of an Nd:YAG laser and vice versa (Fig. 3-1).[3]

Patients do not have the protection of hospital accreditation procedures when the surgeon plans to use lasers outside the hospital in an office setting. Furthermore, surgeons do not have clear-cut guidelines for safe use of lasers outside hospital operating rooms and treatment rooms. For office use, therefore, surgeons must be doubly sure that their training in laser surgery and their adherence to strict safety procedures are complete and thoroughly documented.

INFORMED CONSENT

If the surgeon plans to operate with the laser, he should inform the patient and obtain the patient's consent. The surgeon must be ready to answer the patient's questions, which range from basic to sophisticated. In answering these questions and obtaining the patient's

Laser Privilege Form

Name_____ Signature_____

Title/Position _____

Laser Course:
    Name _____

    Program Director_____

    Location_____

    Date _____

    Hours_____

In House Experience:
    Procedure _____

    Date _____

    By _____
             (signature of observer)

    Procedure _____

    Date _____

    By _____
             (signature of observer)

    Procedure _____

    Date _____

    By _____
             (signature of observer)

Laser Type_____

Laser Privileges:_____

Approval

Date	Departmental Chairman
Date	Chairman of Laser Safety Committee
Date	Executive Board of the Medical Staff
Date	Ethics and Credentials Committee

Figure 3–1. Sample laser privilege form. This form records instruction in laser surgery, in-house experience, and approval by hospital authorities. This degree of documentation and approval protects patients from being treated by inexperienced operators and ensures that the surgeon has laser skills.

consent, the surgeon must have a clear understanding of the reasons for laser use and the goals to be achieved. In general, the CO_2 laser functions as a scalpel. The surgeon should explain to patients that the advantages of CO_2 laser include increased accuracy, improved hemostasis, and sterilization of the operating field, but he should also inform the patient of the potential hazards. If the CO_2 laser is to be used for arthroscopy, ablation of tissue, vaporization of cement and plastic, or tissue repairs, the patient must understand that the laser will be used as well as the benefits and potential complications of its use. The patient should also be informed of the alternatives to laser use. It should be noted that the FDA, having found the CO_2 laser to be substantially equivalent to electrosurgical equipment in surgery, has approved almost all uses for CO_2 lasers. Most hospitals and surgeons have not devised a special consent form for CO_2 laser use; however, the space describing the operation on the operative permits and consent forms must be filled out appropriately to show that the surgeon has explained laser use to the patient.

In contrast to routine CO_2 laser usage, the Nd:YAG laser, dye lasers, and other types of lasers have had far less use in orthopaedics, so this type of surgery must be considered innovative if not experimental. Informed consent under these circumstances may require completion of more than a routine hospital form. This is especially so if the surgeon is involved in a protocol and is performing surgery under an IDE issued by the FDA. A consent form for this type of surgery, in which patients are placed on an experimental protocol, requires approval by the Institutional Review Board of the hospital before being submitted to the FDA. If the surgeon believes, however, that use of one of these devices is in the patient's best interest and that the operation with the laser will provide for the best outcome, a special consent form need not be utilized. A standard informed consent that outlines the risks and benefits suffices.

EYE PROTECTION

All personnel in the operating room must use protective eye wear because accidental exposure to the concentrated electromagnetic energy in the laser beam can inflict severe injury to the cornea and retina. Should this occur with the CO_2 laser, the injury will consist primarily of scleral or corneal burns because the CO_2 laser beam vaporizes the water in these tissues on contact. Accidental exposure to the Nd:YAG or argon laser, however, will produce a much more serious injury. These lasers tend to pass through the clear cornea to be absorbed by the lens of the eye. Cataracts can result from this type of laser injury. Retinal tissue, which is highly pigmented, readily absorbs the laser energy of visible light. Absorption of these lasers by the retina causes deep thermal necrosis with retinal scarring, which results in blindness. Figure 3-2 summarizes eye injuries caused by various types of lasers.

Several factors determine the appropriate eyewear to be utilized in protection of the eyes during laser use. The most important consideration in this regard is the optical density of the eyewear and its ability to attenuate the potentially damaging wavelengths emitted by the laser. In the case of a CO_2 laser, clear glass, transparent plastic, or quartz glasses with side protectors provide satisfactory eye protection (Fig. 3-3). In the case of the Nd:YAG laser, protective glasses with blue green lenses are required; for argon lasers, glasses with orange yellow lenses are necessary (Fig. 3-4). The use of lasers in a closed system such as arthroscopic surgery (in which operating-

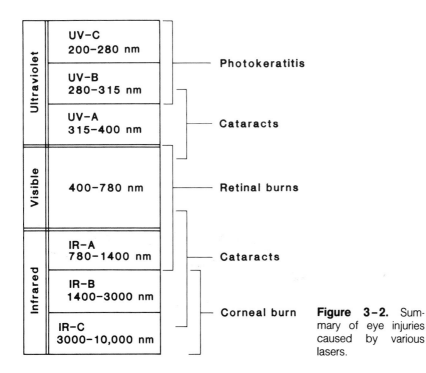

Figure 3-2. Summary of eye injuries caused by various lasers.

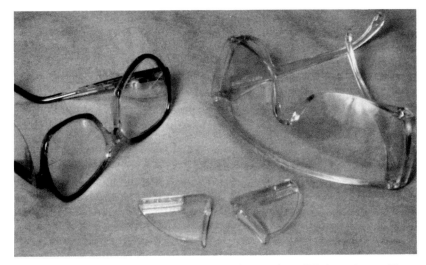

Figure 3–3. Clear glass or plastic protects the eye from CO_2 laser burns. There should be side protectors on the glasses and goggles to prevent laser energy reflected off shiny surfaces from striking the cornea.

room personnel are not exposed to the laser beam) might be considered an exception to the rule that the protective glasses be used at all times. The opportunity for accidental exposure does exist, however, so for complete safety, the glasses should always be worn (Fig. 3–5).

Other considerations in determining the appropriate eyewear are ability to transmit visible light, comfort and fit, strength of materials, and durability of the absorbing medium so that the eyewear remains safe as long as it is in use.

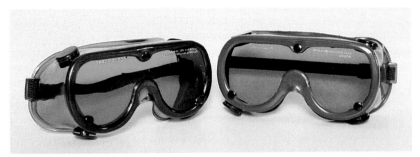

Figure 3–4. Nd:YAG lasers require green glasses or goggles, and argon lasers require orange or red glasses or goggles for protection.

In providing for eye protection, the surgical team must utilize other precautionary measures. The operating room must have limited access to prevent unprotected personnel or personnel not familiar with laser safety and usage from entering. The operating room should have a sign posted at the door showing that the laser is in use and that protective eyewear should be worn. In addition, the warning should state what type of laser is being used and what type of eyewear is required (Fig. 3–6). When the laser is in use, the beam should never be directed against shiny polished surfaces, because a reflected laser beam can inadvertently injure a person in the operating room. For this reason, the surgical instruments should be black-

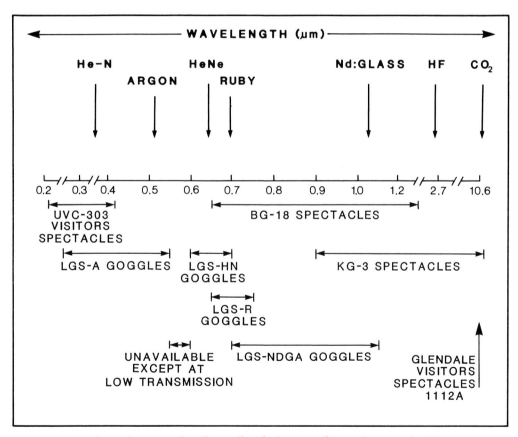

Figure 3–5. Different laser wavelengths on the electromagnetic spectrum require different types of eye protection. This figure shows what type of eye protection is required for the various lasers.

ened or shiny surfaces dulled. The diffuse reflection from such surfaces sharply decreases the radiant exposure of the eye, whereas the "specular reflection" from mirrorlike surfaces causes an intra-beam viewing of the laser, which may cause serious eye damage. When working around polished orthopaedic implants, the reflective surfaces should be covered with wet towels or sponges. Finally, the laser should be switched off or on standby when lasing is not in progress, and the operator's foot should never be on the foot pedal when not in use. If other instruments requiring foot pedals are utilized during the operation, the laser pedal should be on the opposite side of the table. The other instruments should be activated by an assistant, so that the surgeon will not inadvertently step on the laser pedal and send the laser beam into an unintended target.

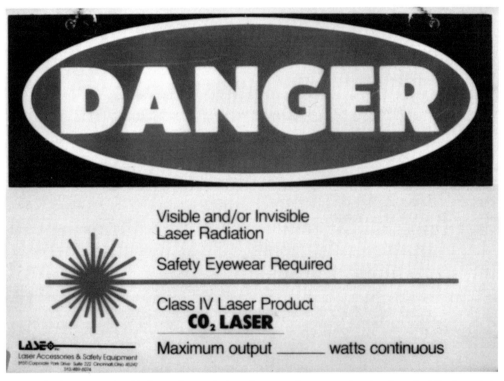

Figure 3-6. A sign should always be posted on the operating room door to show that the laser is in use and that protective eye wear should be worn. The sign should indicate what type of laser is being used so that those entering will know what kind of eye wear is required.

The patient's eyes must also be covered and protected with moist pads during laser use if the patient is being operated on with a general anesthetic. If spinal anesthesia or local anesthesia is being used, the patient should wear protective glasses, the color and optical density of the glasses being determined by the type of laser.[1,2,10]

FIRE PREVENTION

Operating-room fires are potential complications of laser use, and precautions must be taken by the anesthetists and surgeons to avoid them. The extreme heat of the laser can ignite flammable anesthetic gases, so anesthesiologists should not use these agents on a patient having laser surgery. Endotracheal tubes present two major hazards. First, certain types of endotracheal tubes are flammable. Polyvinyl chloride and rubber tubes can be ignited by the heat of the lasing, and the burning tube and its combustion can cause massive tissue destruction in the lungs and tracheobronchial tree. For this reason, in laser surgery performed on the neck and cervical spine, anesthetists should select tubes that do not burn. Polyvinyl chloride can ignite at 149°F and rubber at 240°F, whereas Silastic tubes ignite at temperatures above 700°F. Silastic tubes or metal tubes, therefore, are preferred when laser surgery is done in this anatomic area.[9,10]

A second potential complication with endotracheal tubes is perforation of the tube by the laser beam. If an oxygen-rich gas mixture is present in the tube at the time of perforation, a flame-out can occur, causing searing of the lungs with the potential for the death of the patient. To prevent this catastrophe, the anesthesiologist should use gas mixtures containing less that 40% oxygen and avoid the use of combustible agents such as nitrous oxide. The endotracheal tube can be coated or wrapped with a protective, partially reflective covering. The surgeon should avoid prolonged lasing of the area of the endotracheal tube and direct the beam parallel to the tube and not directly at it. If a fire, however brief, should occur, the anesthetist should stop the oxygen flow at once and remove the tube. The patient should be bronchoscoped and reintubated, and the tracheobronchial tree thoroughly assessed for any damage. Tracheotomy may be necessary, and steroids and antibiotics almost certainly will be required.[9,10]

The intense heat of the laser can also damage tissue if the surgeon does not exercise certain precautions. Prolonged continuous lasing in a small area can raise the local temperature high enough to cause extensive damage. This is especially true if the tissue exposed to the laser can transmit heat well. Bone, for example, conducts heat very rapidly and becomes very hot when directly exposed to the laser beam.

In addition, if the power density is set too low, the laser might heat the tissues rather than vaporize them. If the temperature of the tissue rises far enough, the products of vaporization can also be heated — even up to the critical point of igniting. A brief flame-out of the laser plume, therefore, suggests that the surgeon should adjust the power density or focus the beam of the laser to raise the power density high enough to cause vaporization instead of local heating.

One can also avoid these problems by using the laser in short bursts, cooling the tissues with periodic saline spray, and using the highest power density possible for as short a period of time as possible to avoid heating the surrounding tissues. Moist towels should be sutured or clipped to the skin edges before turning on the laser, and the saline spray should be used liberally during the lasing to keep the towels and wound moist.

SMOKE EVACUATION

Lasers currently in use achieve their effect by quickly heating intracellular and extracellular water above 100°C and vaporizing it. All cells containing the water swell and almost instantaneously explode. The water vapor and carbon residue are released by this process to produce the smoke occasionally referred to as the *laser plume*. The laser plume released during the use of a CO_2 laser contains particles with a median diameter of 0.31 μ. These particles are smaller in size than red blood cells, for example, and they are too small to be filtered by the average surgical mask; therefore, unless an efficient vacuum system is used, operating surgical teams will inhale large numbers of the particles. Because viruses and other DNA molecules are possibly carried on the particles in the laser plume, there is some concern that the personnel in the operating room have a hazardous exposure to papilloma viruses or AIDS viruses. Furthermore, prolonged inhalation of carbon particles in the plume may expose personnel to mutagenic smoke much like that noted in passive inhalation of cigarette smoke. The question of DNA molecules in the laser plume, however, is not yet clarified, and the danger may be over-stated, because the DNA molecules may well be unbonded into harmless fragments of carbon, nitrogen, and oxygen by lasing. The intense heat of the laser sterilizes tissue by vaporizing bacterial organisms as well as the cells in the target tissues. The laser plume, therefore, is probably bacteriologically sterile.[5]

The chemical products of vaporization of laser use may also be hazardous.[4,8] In the removal of polymethlymethacrylate (PMMA) during total joint revision, the heat of the laser breaks down the PMMA into its monomeric form, which is then sublimated into gaseous by-products such as formaldehyde, carbon monoxide, and hydrocyanic acid.[7] These by-products are detectable in the plume, but when an efficient vacuum system is used, it is virtually all removed from the operating-room air breathed by the surgical team. In our experiments, we could detect only 8.6 ppm of unidentifiable hydrocarbons in the air breathed by the surgical team during the PMMA lasing when the vacuum system was in use. This level is well within safe limits as recommended by OSHA (see Chapt. 7).

To avoid the possible hazards of exposure to the laser plume, the operating team must use a powerful smoke-evacuation vacuum system at all times during lasing. The system should be vented to the outside, and there should be frequent maintenance checks as well as replacement of the filters in the system on a regular basis. If the vacuum system is used conscientiously, the laser plume is barely visible and there is no odor of smoke during lasing.[4,7,8]

OTHER SAFETY CONSIDERATIONS

Other concerns about use of lasers relate primarily to safety considerations for powerful electrical devices. Personnel working in the operating room should not stand in wet spots or puddles when they are operating any electrical device; injuries, burns, and electrocution have been reported. If the protective panels are removed from the laser while it is in use, burns or fires can occur. To avoid the chance of spilling liquid into the electrical system, the laser top should not be used as a prep tray or coffee table. Finally, the laser and the vacuum system tend to be noisy. Conversations and radio playing can add to the cacophony, which may distract some people operating the lasers.

REFERENCES

1. American National Standards for the Safe Use of Lasers. (ANSI 2136.1) New York, American National Standards Institute, 1986
2. Bohignan GM: Lasers in medicine and surgery: The other issues. JAMA 256:909–910, 1982
3. Baggish MS: Education of the laser surgeon. Lasers Surg Med 5:485–489, 1985
4. Choy DS, Kaminow IP, Kaplan M et al: Experimental Nd:YAG laser disintegration of methylmethacrylate: analysis of gaseous products. Clin Orthop 215:287–288, 1987
5. Clinical Laser Monthly 5, No. 4:41–44, 1987
6. Council on Scientific Affairs. Lasers in medicine and surgery. JAMA 256, No. 7:900–907, 1986
7. Ganel A, Farine I, Horoszynski H: Bone cement melted by a laser beam: analysis. Lasers Electro-Optics 1:12–13, 1981
8. Knoll DA, Morris MD, Norton ML: Hazards of degradation of methlymethacrylate. Anesthesia 61, No 1:115–116, 1984
9. Mahr RM, McDonnell BC, Unger M et al: Safety considerations and safety protocol for laser surgery. Surg Clin North Am 64, No. 5:851–859, 1984
10. Rockwell RJ: Hazard levels, safety procedures, and standards for Nd:YAG laser surgery. In Breedlowe B, Schwartz D (eds): Clinical Lasers: Expert Strategies for Practical & Profitable Management, pp 50–51. Atlanta, American Health Consultants, 1984
11. Standards of Practice for the Use of Lasers in Medicine and Surgery. Wasau, American Society for Laser Medicine and Surgery, 1984

4

Laser Surgery in Other Disciplines: Physics, Applications, and New Horizons

Howard A. Zaren
Joaquin Sariego
Bernard Sigel

Advances in medical technology in the past 25 years have been paralleled by an increasing sophistication on the part of the general public concerning the applicability of such technology. For this reason, lasers have captured the attention and interest of both the medical and lay communities as they become a more vital part of the medical armamentarium. Not long ago, the laser as considered a curiosity. Today, however, it has become a routine treatment tool in all fields of medicine. Current uses of lasers range from the treatment of hemorrhoids and arthritis to heart disease and cancer. Already a mainstay of treatment in ophthalmology, otolaryngology, dermatology, and gynecology, the laser is finding a vital place in other specialties as well, including general surgery and orthopaedics. As a result of these developments, it is essential to understand the background of the laser as a medical tool, as well as the basic principles underlying its action. This chapter briefly describes these basic principles and then summarizes the myriad of nonorthopaedic uses of the laser.

LASER PHYSICS

A number of devices used in patient care require little technical knowledge other than a general understanding of the principles of application. The laser, however, is different because it is a powerful instrument that is capable of causing a great deal of destruction or damage; therefore, it is essential that surgeons using the laser have some basic understanding of laser technology. In addition, a basic understanding of the principles of physics that govern laser technology will enable the surgeon to assess new applications more competently, to evaluate laser effects more critically, and to use this powerful tool safely.

Laser is an acronym for light amplification by the stimulated emission of radiation. Each word used in forming this acronym relates to a basic concept of physics necessary for an understanding of laser light; these concepts are summarized in the following sections.

Properties of Light (*L*ASER)

Light is a form of electromagnetic energy that can be visible or invisible to the human eye depending on its wavelength on the electromagnetic spectrum. All forms of transmitted energy, in a very broad sense, may be viewed as light. Many questions about the nature of electromagnetic energy still need to be answered. At the present time, scientists describe light using both wave and particle theories of physics. The wave theory views light as a wave similar to a water wave. These waves are characterized by amplitude, frequency, and wavelength. The vertical height of a wave is called *amplitude* and is related to the intensity of the light. The *frequency* of a wave is the number of vibrations per second, and is expressed in hertz. The distance from one peak or valley to the next is defined as a *wavelength*. Wavelength and frequency determine the energy level of the light and how it is categorized on the electromagnetic-energy spectrum. The longer wavelengths of the spectrum are of lower energy and fall into the infrared zone; they include microwaves, televisions, and AM radios. Shorter wavelengths have higher energy and include ultraviolet light and x-rays.

The laser is a beam of intense light that emits energy in wavelengths that range from near ultraviolet to near infrared. The energy level of the laser beam and its position on the electromagnetic spectrum are determined by wavelength and frequency. Whether the laser light is visible or invisible depends on the medium used to generate light. Argon, helium, neon, and ruby are the most popular visible light lasers. The Nd:YAG laser generates invisible laser light at a wavelength of 1.06 μm, which is in the near infrared region of the electromagnetic spectrum. the CO_2 laser is characterized by a very long wavelength compared with visible light and is in the far infrared region of the electromagnetic spectrum.

The theory that light is composed of particles was espoused as far back as Newton. In the 20th century, the word *quanta* was introduced by Einstein to describe the particles of energy composing light. In the 1920s, the word *photon* came into use to define the energy in particles of light. Einstein theorized that light traveled in streams of massless particles called photons, and each of these photons carried a quantum of energy associated with a specific wavelength of light.[9] Experiments have been performed that prove both the wave and particle theories; however, neither theory fully explains all the phenomena of light or of other forms of electromagnetic energy.

Laser Light

The following properties distinguish laser light from plain, white light:

1. It is monochromatic; that is, all the light produced by the laser is one wavelength or color.
2. It is directional; that is, the beam from the laser does not expand as quickly as other light and will not spread out like ordinary light beams.
3. It is coherent; that is, the waves of light are in phase with each other, and the crests and troughs of wavelengths are lined up with each other and coincide. Because many wavelengths comprise ordinary light, they cannot be generated together nor stay together as they travel. Ordinary light is therefore considered incoherent.

These properties of light correspond to the "L" in the acronym *laser* and are the special properties of laser light.

Amplification (LASER)

Amplification identifies the final coordination of light energy that is emitted as a unified, efficient beam from the laser device. This occurs when the wavelengths of light energy are in phase; in other words, the troughs and peaks of each wave line up and amplify each other as they travel through the laser medium toward the transparent mirror located at one end of the laser where they may be emitted as a beam of coherent laser light. Only a small portion of the total energy created within the medium (*i.e.*, CO_2, Nd:YAG, crystal neon) is emitted as a coordinated beam of light; most of the energy is emitted as spontaneous energy in the form of heat. In comparison to incoherent light, laser light can deliver high amounts of energy over long distances reliably. The resulting laser light will be monochromatic, directional, and coherent.

Stimulated Emission (LASER)

Stimulated emission occurs when the atoms in the laser medium are charged with energy from an external source, resulting in the emission of photons from the excited electrons. A review of physicist Max Planck's quantum theory will provide a basis for an understanding of this process. According to this theory, electrons in orbits of varying energy levels surround the nucleus located at the center of the atom. The electrons traveling in the orbit closest to the nucleus are in the lowest energy level. Most atoms tend to remain at the lowest energy level, which is called the *ground state.* An electron will jump from a low energy orbit into a higher energy orbit, when it obtains energy from an outside source. The electron, however, remains in the excited state a fraction of a second and then returns to a lower energy level, at which point it releases its energy in the form of a photon. The emitted photon will have the same wavelength as the photon absorbed by the electron. This release of energy is called *spontaneous emission.*

In the 1920s, Einstein established a theory called *stimulated emission*, which explained what happens when an electron already in an excited state absorbs energy from an outside source. Before Einstein's theory, it was assumed that an excited electron would jump to a higher level if stimulated by another photon. Einstein, however, theorized that if a photon of a specific wavelength hits an excited electron with the same wavelength, the stimulated electron would emit a photon and return to a lower energy level rather than absorb the incident photon. Consequently, two photons of the same wavelength are released to travel on their way. He further theorized that these released photons would stimulate neighboring electrons of the same wavelength to radiate photons, precipitating a chain reaction of photon emission called stimulated emission. This coordination of waves then results in the unified emission of laser light. The stimulated-emission process creates another of the special properties of the laser light called *coherence.* When one photon stimulates emission of another, the new photon begins life in the same phase as the photon that stimulated it. When all the photons are in phase, they are said to be coherent.

Because most atoms try to be in the lowest energy state, spontaneous emission — with electrons returning to ground state — is more natural than stimulated emission. In order to generate a sufficient number of excited electrons to achieve stimulated emission, an out-side source of energy is required to rouse the resting electrons into a more energized state. When the outside source generates more excited electrons than resting electrons, this state is called *population inversion.* In order to produce the stimulated emission required for creation of a laser beam, it is necessary to induce a population inversion.

Radiation (LASER)

Laser light is a form of electromagnetic radiation. All electromagnetic radiation travels at the speed of light, and the wavelength of the radiation is the determining factor in whether or not this electromagnetic energy is visible or invisible. Laser light can be either visible or invisible. Argon, helium–neon, and ruby lasers, for example, are visible; excimer and Nd:YAG lasers are invisible.

Because shorter wavelengths have a higher frequency, they contain more energy per photon than longer wavelengths of energy. Excimer lasers are located in the near ultraviolet end of the electromagnetic spectrum and therefore have a shorter wavelength and more energy than the CO_2 laser.

Laser Components

All lasers, regardless of laser style, size, or application, contain four primary components. These components include the active medium, the excitation mechanism, the feedback mechanism, and the output coupler. The generation of laser light takes place in the active medium, which can be a solid, liquid, a gas, or a semiconductor material. The laser light is generated by exciting the atoms, molecules, or ions of the medium. The properties of the medium determine the wavelength and other characteristics of the laser light that is produced.

The feedback mechanism includes two mirrors — the reflectance mirror, which is 100% reflective, and the output coupler, which is a partially transparent mirror. Johnson states that "these mirrors are specially designed for the laser wavelengths and consist of a glass based material with very thin, dielectric coating with vapor deposits on the glass for reflective surfaces."[1] When photons hit the reflectance mirror, they are redirected back into the medium, where they stimulate electrons to emit photons. The coherent light resulting from this process of stimulated emission is transmitted through the partially transparent output coupler in the form of a laser beam.

The excitation mechanism is an external source of energy that activates the electrons in the laser medium. In solid-state lasers, an intense light source is used to excite the medium. A flash lamp, for example, is used to excite a YAG crystal. Excitation in a gas medium is produced by passing an electric current through the gas.

The laser unit consists of a long resonator tube that contains the laser medium. The mirrors are positioned on either end of the tube.

APPLICATIONS

The first functioning laser was developed in 1960, and investigators immediately began experimenting with various medical applications.[2,6] Not until 1970, however, were effective focusing and control mechanisms developed that allowed the laser to be used as a clinical tool. The first such laser to be used in this role was the CO_2 laser.[7] Several years later, the Nd:YAG and argon ion lasers were applied clinically. Initially, the Nd:YAG laser was used endoscopically to treat bleeding gastrointestinal lesions;[8] the argon laser was used to treat dermatologic disorders.[9] Since then, the uses of these types of lasers have expanded to encompass a broad range of conditions and disorders that are amenable to extirpative and palliative uses of the laser.

Early lasers and the CO_2 and Nd:YAG lasers in use today are classified as thermal lasers because their action depends upon the dissipation of energy as heat. This process is discussed in the section on laser physics in this chapter. More recently, nonthermal laser technology, termed *photodynamic therapy*, has been developed that allows the laser to be used effectively in a diagnostic role as well as a therapeutic role.[10] This is discussed in more detail in the section on laser physics in this chapter.

In short, in the past 25 years, laser technology has made tremendous advances. Clearly, lasers are no longer technologic curiosities; they have become invaluable tools in the armamentarium of modern medical and surgical science.

Types of Lasers

Theoretically, the number of potential laser systems is as limitless as the number of wavelengths found to be emitted by a host of solid, liquid, and gas media. Realistically, however, only a few of these wavelengths have been found to have clinical usefulness. The major lasers in use today are based upon the emission of energy wavelengths from certain standard compounds. Specifically, most clinical systems are based upon CO_2, Nd:YAG, argon, or certain other rare gases as laser media.

CO_2 Laser

The CO_2 laser, the first laser developed for clinical use, generates energy at a wavelength of 10.6 μm, which falls in the infrared region of the electromagnetic spectrum. The medium is actually a mixture of gases containing CO_2, helium, and nitrogen. Carbon dioxide is the active component, and the other gases facilitate the transfer of vibrational energy.

Although the CO_2 laser does not penetrate tissue as deeply as other types of lasers (*e.g.*, the Nd:YAG laser), it vaporizes tissue readily because the laser energy is absorbed rapidly by the tissue.[10] In addition, pulse duration can be varied with the CO_2 laser so as to effect minimal thermal diffusion from the treated area and, thus, cause only minimal tissue damage.[11] These characteristics make the CO_2 laser a useful tool in ablation and coagulation of superficial and dermatologic lesions.

Unfortunately, the delivery system is somewhat cumbersome, necessitating an articulated arm in order to transmit the beam to the target. Although more streamlined delivery systems are being developed, no effective and practical method has been developed to transmit the CO_2 beam through flexible fibers. Until such a system is widely available, the usefulness of the CO_2 laser intra-abdominally and endoscopically is limited.

Nd:YAG Laser

Neodymium (Nd), which produces a wavelength of 1.06 μm (near infrared), was developed as a laser medium as early as 1961.[12] Coupled with glass, however, this early laser was difficult to operate continuously because of the low thermal conductivity of the glass. Later, however, neodymium was combined with yttrium aluminum garnet (YAG) to create a much more effective system. This Nd:YAG laser has excellent tissue penetration compared with the CO_2 laser. In turn, because the Nd:YAG laser does not vaporize tissue as readily as the CO_2 laser, the former affects a much larger volume of tissue than the latter. The Nd:YAG laser can therefore better coagulate surrounding vessels and tissue.

The Nd:YAG laser may be operated in a continuous or pulsed

fashion that can deliver energy of greater intensity to disrupt cell membranes and other structures.

Because of its good tissue penetration and coagulation capacity, as well as its ability to be transmitted via flexible fiberoptics, the Nd:YAG has become the standard laser used endoscopically. It has been used during bronchoscopy, esophagoscopy, colonoscopy, and laparoscopy for tumor coagulation and ablation.

Argon

Argon is only one of several gaseous ions that has been used as a laser medium; however, it has become one of the few to enjoy widespread clinical applicability. Developed in 1964,[13] it initially was used primarily in the field of ophthalmology.

The fundamental action of ion lasers in general (and the argon laser in particular) is dependent upon the ionization of the active gaseous medium by high electrical-current densities passed through the gas. This involves a considerable dissipation of heat; therefore, air- and water-cooled systems are necessary.

The light emitted by the argon laser is in the blue green region of the visible spectrum and has a wavelength of 0.488 μm. This laser has an intermediate level of light transmission between the CO_2 and Nd:YAG lasers and thus causes a degree of tissue injury somewhere between the two types of laser applications.[10]

The argon laser may be used alone or in conjunction with a dye laser as a component of photodynamic therapy.

Excimer Laser

Excimer lasers utilize the media of rare gas halides. Each gas has a defined wavelength of emitted energy. The most commonly used gases are krypton fluoride (0.193 μm) and xenon fluoride (0.35 μm). All of these wavelengths lie within the ultraviolet portion of the electromagnetic spectrum. Although still a tool of largely unknown potential, the excimer laser may find applicability in a wide range of surgical and medical fields.

Laser Applications

Lasers of all types are now widely used in all branches of medicine and surgery. Naturally, specific lasers have specific functions within a given subspecialty, and these functions are based upon the unique characteristics and physical properties of the various systems.

Head and Neck

The primary surgical laser utilized in otolaryngology is the CO_2 laser. First applied in the early 1970s,[14] the high water and tissue absorptive capacity of the CO_2 laser has made it a useful tool in head and neck surgery. Although it is unable to be transmitted through a fiberoptic system, the CO_2 beam may be focused easily using an articulated arm. It has been used to treat a variety of head and neck lesions.

Using a wide-angle laryngoscope and suspension laryngoscopy, the CO_2 laser may be used in conjunction with an operating microscope for laryngeal surgery. This technique is effective in the treatment of laryngeal stenosis from scars or webs. Vocal-cord nodules or polyps may be treated with a low-power CO_2 beam as well.

Another use of the CO_2 laser is for arytenoidectomy in patients with bilateral vocal-cord paralysis that is causing respiratory stridor.[15] This technique may be used to avoid an open laryngeal procedure or the need for a permanent tracheotomy.

The CO_2 laser may also be used to perform excisional biopsies of cancers of the true vocal cords. This excision can also be performed in conjunction with the operating microscope.

Finally, the CO_2 laser beam can now be delivered via recently developed flexible fibers and no longer needs to be coupled to a rigid bronchoscope for treatment of lesions of the tracheobronchial tree.[16] This technique is used primarily for treatment of recurrent respiratory papillomatosis and palliation from obstructing tracheal lesions.

Much more effective for the treatment of obstructing tracheobronchial lesions, however, is the Nd:YAG laser,[17] which has the advantage of providing better coagulation owing to its deeper penetration. Also, it may be used through a fiberoptic bronchoscope for better visualization. The less predictable depth of tissue penetration makes the Nd:YAG laser more suitable for tissue ablation and coagulation, as opposed to biopsy, for which the CO_2 laser may be applicable.

The role of the argon laser has been limited to photodynamic therapy of recurrent or early metastatic cancers of the head and neck. This technique is in more detail later in this chapter.

Gynecology

The first uses of laser technology in gynecology involved the treatment of superficial and cervical lesions with the CO_2 laser. This system is still commonly used, in conjunction with colposcopy, to

43

treat intra-epithelial neoplasia (or carcinoma in situ) of the cervix. Mounted on a colposcope, the CO_2 laser accurately achieves ablation, excision, or vaporization of cervical lesions; is commonly used to perform cervical conization; and is usually an effective treatment for carcinoma in situ. Because approximately 99% of these lesions extend no further than 4 mm from the surface into the cervical crypt,[18] excision of this volume of tissue is within the capabilities of the CO_2 laser. Cure rates using this technique are greater than 97%.[19]

A second use of the CO_2 laser is in the treatment of vulvar and vaginal lesions. If the neoplasm is not invasive and is documented to be intra-epithelial, superficial laser vulvectomy may be performed easily and usually without the need for a skin graft. Similar power densities may be used to ablate condyloma acuminata. Complications in these procedures are rare, and scarring is generally minimal.

Lasers have also been used intra-abdominally with great success for a number of indications. In the treatment of infertility, for example, the CO_2 laser has been very useful intraoperatively because of limited tissue injury, rapid healing, minimal scarring, and adequate superficial hemostasis. This laser may be used in a microscope or hand-held system for lysis of adhesions, vaporization of endometriosis, neosalpingostomy, resection of ectopic pregnancy, tubal reanastomosis, and myomectomy.[20]

More recently, lasers have also been used laparoscopically with great success.[21] Both CO_2 and Nd:YAG lasers may now be employed in this fashion, and each type has specific uses. As mentioned previously, the CO_2 laser may be employed for procedures necessitating accurate focusing and minimal scarring; for example, it is well suited for enterolysis and procedures upon the tubes and ovaries. The Nd:YAG laser, on the other hand, is most useful for tumor ablation and tissue coagulation. In addition, it has been used successfully during laparoscopy to treat recurrences of intraperitoneal tumors or implants; during hysteroscopy, it has been effective in intrauterine surgery.[22] Finally, the argon laser, which is absorbed well by melanin and hemoglobin, has been used in the treatment of pelvic endometriosis.[23]

Dermatology

Although various types of lasers have been used to treat dermatologic disorders, the CO_2 and argon lasers are the most widely used. The CO_2 laser is especially well suited for dermatologic disorders because its small depth penetration and minimal scatter enable effective localization of an area of destruction, which results in minimal damage to adjacent tissue.

The CO_2 laser may be used as a cutting or as an ablative instrument. The theoretical advantage of the laser as a "thermal knife" is that it cuts and permits hemostasis simultaneously. In reality, however, no clear advantage has been shown in terms of reduced operating time, diminished blood loss, or wound healing.[10] The exception to this is the patient with a coagulopathy or in whom an excessively large vascular field is being treated. Such a procedure would include treatment of rhinophyma, excision of scalp tumors, and scalp reductions. In these cases, use of the CO_2 laser may be desirable to minimize blood loss.

As an ablative tool, the CO_2 laser is commonly used to remove warts, tattoos, sublingual keratosis, epidermal nevi, and a variety of other lesions. Also, a number of vascular skin lesions, including port wine stains, cherry angiomas, pyogenic granulomas, and angiokeratomas, respond well to CO_2 laser therapy.

The argon laser also is useful in treating dermatologic disorders. Its absorption is selective but also dependent upon pigmentation of the epidermis (*i.e.*, absorption increases with increased pigmentation). Also, argon light is preferentially absorbed by hemoglobin, melanin, and other dark skin pigments. The argon laser, therefore, is useful predominantly for the treatment of pigmented lesions such as port wine stains, hemangiomas, and tattoos. Results with port wine stains are excellent in 8% to 10% of patients and good to fair in 70% of patients.[24]

The Nd:YAG laser has limited usefulness in cutaneous surgery because penetration into tissue is deep and scatter is high; however, it has been used in treatment of deep vascular lesions and in coagulation necrosis of malignant skin tumors.

Urology

Various lasers have been found useful in the treatment of specific urologic disorders. As mentioned previously, properties of the CO_2 laser make it an excellent tool for the treatment of condyloma acuminata, urethral strictures, and superficial lesions (*e.g.*, erythroplasia of Queyrat). The argon laser has found some applicability in the treatment of hemangiomatous lesions, small papillary tumors, and arteriovenous malformations.

The most versatile laser available for urologic use is the Nd:YAG laser. It has been used with good results in the treatment of invasive squamous cell carcinoma of the penis, although clinical experience is limited in the United States. A more common application of the urologic laser in the United States is in the treatment of superficial bladder tumors, which may be successfully ablated during cystoscopy. This application is usually limited to patients with previous histories of superficial, papillary, and transitional cell carcinoma of the bladder; normal or low-grade malignant cells on voided cytology; papillary tumor at cystoscopy; and tumor less than 3 cm in size.[25] Using these criteria, local recurrence is as low as 4% to 5%, although tumor recurrence in remote areas of the bladder may still be as high as 37%.[26] This compares favorably, however, to electrocoagulation therapy of these tumors. The Nd:YAG laser has also been used to treat invasive bladder cancer, although these results have been less encouraging. Finally, the Nd:YAG laser has been used for ureteric and kidney lesions; however, most reports of such usage are preliminary or investigational.

Gastroenterology

The most widely known and studied application of the Nd:YAG laser is in the treatment of gastrointestinal disorders. Specifically, some of the earliest reports of the use of lasers in medicine involved the endoscopic control of gastrointestinal hemorrhage using the Nd:YAG laser. This has been a particularly useful tool because of its deep tissue penetration and effective coagulation of vessels and surrounding tissue. Angiodysplasias of the upper and lower gastrointestinal tract, as well as Mallory-Weiss tears of the esophagus, may be controlled with the Nd:YAG laser. Also, bleeding gastric and duodenal ulcers are amenable to laser hemostasis. In acute ulcer bleeding, 82% of cases are controlled, with a 30% re-bleeding rate. In chronic ulcer bleeding, 95% of cases are controlled, with a 6% re-bleeding rate.[27] The argon laser may also be used for hemostasis of gastrointestinal bleeding. In fact, its greater absorption and lesser penetration may produce less transmural damage than the Nd:YAG laser. Nevertheless, its greater availability and familiarity have made the Nd:YAG the predominant laser in the treatment of this condition.

A second major area of application for the laser is in the ablation and resection of obstructing or bleeding tumors of the gastroinestinal tract. Once again, the Nd:YAG laser has been the predominant system utilized. With obstructing esophageal tumors, use of the Nd:YAG laser via the endoscope can result in successful resection and palliation in 75% to 95% of cases, with a procedure-related mortality rate of 5%.[28,30]

Similarly favorable results have been reported in the treatment of colon and rectal lesions. Large, sessile, villous polyps of the colon can be resected with results that are, at least, equivalent to electrosnare techniques via the colonoscope. Multiple investigators have also reported that the Nd:YAG laser used during colonoscopy has achieved successful palliation of inoperable lesions of the colon and rectum in numerous cases.[31,32] Although perforations are uncommon, delayed stenosis may be a late complication in a minority of patients treated with this technique; nevertheless, laser palliation is a viable alternative to permanent colostomy in those patients with low-lying, unrespectable colorectal lesions.

Laser therapy may also be used in the treatment of hemorrhoids. painful thrombosed hemorrhoids may be effectively excised and coagulated with minimal discomfort and blood loss using any of several laser systems. Once again, lasers with superficial depths of penetration will be unable to coagulate deeper, larger vessels.

Finally, the Nd:YAG laser may be used intraoperatively to ablate peritoneal implants or metastases from a variety of tumors. This may be desirable in those instances in which adequate cytoreductive surgery necessitates the removal of these tumor foci.

Neurosurgery

All three major laser systems (CO_2, Nd:YAG, and argon) have been utilized in the treatment of neurosurgical lesions. The CO_2 laser has been shown to cause a more localized lesion with minimal disruption of the blood–brain barrier; however, the transmission of the CO_2 beam through cerebrospinal fluid is poor, so it is most useful in the treatment of extra-axial brain tumors in sensitive areas in which surrounding damage must be kept to a minimum. The CO_2 laser has limited hemostatic ability; therefore, it must often be coupled with some other system (*e.g.*, Nd:YAG) to achieve adequate coagulation. The Nd:YAG laser will traverse cerebrospinal fluid; thus, intraventricular treatment is possible. Also, because its hemostatic ability is much greater than that of the CO_2 laser, the Nd:YAG laser is much more effective in treating vascular lesions or as an adjunct to CO_2 laser therapy. On the other hand, the deep and distant vascular effects of the Nd:YAG laser render it unsuitable for treatment of spinal tumors. In these cases, the cutting capability of the CO_2 laser and the small spot size of the argon laser make these much safer and more useful modalities.

The argon laser has theoretical advantages over both the Nd:YAG and CO_2 lasers, including small spot size, transmission through cerebrospinal fluid, and good hemostasis. In actuality, studies have not demonstrated clear superiority in practice; nevertheless, the argon laser may be desirable in selective cases.

Vascular Surgery

A relatively new area in which lasers have begun to play a role is vascular surgery. Recent emphasis has been upon ablation of atheromatous plaques.[10] This has been accomplished either by treating the lesions directly by introducing small endoscopes percutaneously, or by pulling a heated metal tip (heated by a laser beam) through the atheroma. As expected, early trials involved high rates of thrombosis and perforation. Using newer techniques, however, complications have been kept to a minimum, allowing laser technology to become more useful in the treatment of vascular lesions. Such techniques may be used not only on peripheral blood vessels, but on coronary arteries as well.

Orthopaedic Surgery

Lasers are being used extensively in orthopaedic surgery as well. Laser energy may be delivered under direct vision or, more specifically, by an arthroscope. This technology has enabled the orthopaedic surgeon to offer noninvasive procedures to a much broader range of patients. It has also expanded the armamentarium of orthopaedic instrumentation.

NEW HORIZONS

As laser technology improves, many new areas of investigation are developing that may, in the long term, greatly expand the clinical uses of lasers. One such area is photodynamic therapy. This modality utilizes a porphyrin compound (a hematoporphyrin derivative) as a tumor photosensitizing agent. After intravenous injection, hematoporphyrin clears from normal tissues within 24 to 48 hours[33]; however, the compound is selectively retained in malignant cells for 10 to 12 days. The compound may be activated by light of a specific wavelength (0.630 μm), and, in the presence of oxygen, produces free radicals that combine with and destroy cell membranes.[34] Photodynamic therapy is thus highly selective for cells that contain the hematoporphyrin compound (*i.e.*, tumor cells). In addition, most tumors (with the exception of those devoid of neovascularity, such as chondrosarcoma) concentrate hematoporphyrin. The compound is activated by light of 0.630 μm that is emitted by a dye laser, which is in turn energized by an argon laser. Photodynamic therapy has many potential benefits. Cutaneous metastases of various tumors can be treated selectively. Superficial bladder tumors and endobronchial lesions may be treated through the cystoscope and bronchoscope, respectively. In addition, because hematoporphyrin is selectively taken up only by tumor cells (visible or microscopic), treatment with the argon dye laser may serve a diagnostic function as well, by localizing as yet unseen metastases.

Although hematoporphyrin does cause temporary skin photosensitization, photodynamic therapy has minimal serious or permanent side-effects on adjacent healthy tissue. As the equipment required to administer photodynamic therapy becomes less cumbersome and more readily available, this technique is likely to enjoy more widespread popularity. Also, as new photosensitizing agents are developed, the range of applications for photodynamic therapy is likely to expand.

Other types of lasers currently available (or being developed) include excimer lasers (see previous section), vapor lasers (including gold and copper), and tunable dye lasers. An example of a vapor laser is the copper–vapor laser, which is a high repitition-rate pulsed laser that emits simultaneously at two wavelengths: 0.51 μm and 0.58 μm. This laser is particularly suited for ocular surgery, especially iridectomy and capsulotomy. Tunable dye lasers utilize pulsed energy with a wide range of energy densities. This allows graded treatment to selectively target specific structures (such as blood vessels) with minimal surrounding damage and scarring. This technique will allow much more specific and individualized treatment for a wide range of conditions.

REFERENCES

1. Johnson JR: Introduction to Laser Biophysics. Orlando, Photon Publishing, 1988
2. Minton JP: The laser in surgery. Am J Surg 151:725–729, 1986
3. Minton JP, Ketchum AS: The laser: A unique oncolytic entity. Am J Surg 108:845–848, 1964
4. Maiman TH: Stimulated optical radiation in ruby. Nature 187:493–494, 1960
5. Minton JP, Ketchum AS, Dearman JR et al: The effects of neodymium laser radiation on two experimental tumor systems. Surg Gynecol Obstet 120:481–478, 1965
6. McGuff PC, Bushnell D, Soroff HS et al: Studies of the surgical applications of lasers. Surg Forum 14:143–145, 1963
7. Pate CKN, McFarlane RA, Faust WL: Selective excitation through vi-

brational energy and optical maser action in N_2CO_2. Physical Rev ABCD 13:617–619, 1964

8. Kiefhaber P, Nath G, Mortij K: Endoscopic control of massive gastrointestinal hemorrhage by irradiational with high power neodymium YAG laser. Prog Surg 15:140–155, 1977

9. Apfelberg DB, Kosek J, Maser MR et al: Histology of port wine stains following argon laser treatment. Br J Plas Surg 32:232–237, 1979

10. Wieman TJ: Lasers and the surgeon. Am J Surg 151:493–500, 1986

11. Walsh JT, Flotte TJ, Anderson RR et al: Pulsed CO_2 laser tissue ablation. Lasers 8:108–118, 1988

12. Smitzer E: Letter: Optical maser action in ND^{3+} in barium crown glass. Physiol Rev 7:444–446, 1961

13. Bridges WB: Letter: Laser oscillation in single ionized argon in the visible spectrum. Appl Physics 5:128–130, 1964

14. Jako GJ: Laser surgery of the vocal cords: An excellent study with carbon dioxide laser on dogs. Laryngoscope 82:2204–2216, 1972

15. Ossoff RH, Sisson GA, Moselle HI et al: Endoscopic laser arytenoidectomy for the treatment of bilateral vocal cord paralysis. Laryngoscope 94:1293–1297, 1984

16. Andres AH, Horowitz SL: Bronchoscopic CO_2 laser surgery. Lasers Surg Med 1:35, 1980

17. Beamis JF, Shapshay SM: Nd:YAG laser therapy for tracheobronchial disorders. Head Neck Surg 75:173–180, 1984

18. Fuller TA (ed): Surgical Lasers: A Clinical Guide, p 67. New York, Macmillan, 1987

19. Fuller TA (ed): Surgical Lasers: A Clinical Guide, p 74. New York, Macmillan, 1987.

20. Fuller TA (ed): Surgical Lasers: A Clinical Guide, p 92. New York, Macmillan, 1987

21. Daniell JF, Brown DH: Carbon dioxide laser laparoscopy: Initial experience in experimental animals and humans. Obstet Gynecol 59:761, 1982

22. Goldrath M, Fuller T, Segal S: Laser photo-vaporization of endometrium for treatment of menorrhagia. Am J Obstet Gynecol 140:14, 1981

23. Kaye WR, Dixon J: Photocoagulation of endometrions by the argon laser through the laparoscope. Obstet Gynecol 62:383, 1983

24. Apfelberg DB, Maser MR, Lash H: Extended clinical use of the argon laser for cutaneous lesions. Arch Dermatol 115:719–721, 1979

25. Fuller TA (ed): Surgical Lasers: A Clinical Guide, p 156. New York, Macmillan, 1987

26. Fuller TA (ed): Surgical Lasers: A Clinical Guide, p 160. New York, Macmillan, 1987

27. Kiefhaber P: Nd:YAG laser surgery statistics. presented at the International Medical Laser Symposium, Detroit, Michigan, March 19–31, 1979

28. Fleischer D, Swak M: Endoscopic Nd:YAG laser therapy as palliation for esophagogastric cancer. Gastroenterology 89:827–831, 1985

29. Lambert R, Sabben G, Chavillon A et al: Results of Nd:YAG laser treatment in epidermoid esophageal cancer. Lasers Surg Med 3:340, 1984

30. Lambert R, Sabben G: Laser therapy for esophageal carcinoma. Lasers Surg Med 3:A253, 1983

31. Lambert R, Sabben G: Laser therapy for colorectal carcinoma. Lasers Surg Med 3:A157, 1983

32. Brunetaud J, Mosquet L, Louche M: Villous adenomas of the rectum: Results of treatment with argon and Nd:YAG lasers. Gastroenterology 89:832–837, 1985

33. Gomer CJ, Dougherty TJ: Determination of [H^3] and [C^4] hematoporphyrin derivative distribution in malignant and normal tissues. Cancer Res 9:146–151, 1979

34. Weishaupt KR, Gomer CJ, Dougherty TJ: Identification of singlet oxygen as the toxic agent in photo inactivation of murine tumor. Cancer Res 36:2326–2329, 1976

BIBLIOGRAPHY

Arndt KA, Noe JM, Northam D et al: Laser therapy: Basic concepts and nomenclature. Am Acad Dermatol 5:649, 1981

Cummins L: Thermal effects of laser radiation on biological tissue. Biophys J 42:99, 1983

Fava G, Emanuelli H, Cascinelli N et al: CO$_2$ lasers: Beam patterns in relation to surgical use. Lasers Surg Med 2:331, 1983

French A, Abela GS, Crea F et al: A comparative study of laser beam characteristics in blood and saline media. Am J Cardiol 55: 1389, 1985

Fuller TA: Fundamentals of lasers in surgery and medicine. In Dixon JS (ed): Surgical Applications of Lasers, pp 11–28. Chicago, Year Book Medical Publishers, 1983

Fuller TA: From source to patient: The Surgical laser delivery system. Lasers Surg Med 3:3–349, 1984

Halldorsson T, Langerholc J: Thermodynamic analysis of laser radiation of biological tissue. Applied Optics 17:3949, 1978

Lipow M: Laser physics made simple. Curr Probl Obstet Gynecol Fertil 9:443, 1986

Lipson SG, Lipson H: Optical Physics, p 268. London, Cambridge University Press, 1969

McKenzie AL, et al: Lasers in surgery and medicine. Phys Med Biol 29:619, 1984

Mester E et al: The biomedical effects of laser application. Lasers Surg Med 5:31, 1985

Rosen DI, Popper LA, Miller MG: Modelling of the laser-induced thermal response and ablation of biological tissue. In Conference on Lasers and

51

Electro Optics: Technical Digest, p 98. Washington, DC, Optical Society of America, 1987

Special Issue on Lasers in Biology and Medicine. IEEE Quan Elect QE20, No. 12: 1984

Stokes LF, Auth DC, Tanaka D et al: Biomedical utility of 1.21 micrometer Nd : YAG laser radiation. IEEE Trans Biomed Eng 28:297, 1981

Welch AJ: The thermal response of laser irradiated tissue. IEEE UJ Quant Elect QE20, No. 12:1471, 1984

Wright VC, Riopelle MA: Laser physics for surgeons. Acta Obstet Gynecol Scand [Suppl] 125:5, 1984

5

Laser – Tissue Interactions and Laser Osteotomy

Henry H. Sherk
Charles Kollmer

The effects of lasers on cartilage, tendon, and other tissues are described in chapters on arthroscopy (Chapt. 9) and tissue welding (Chapt. 8). The effects of lasers on bone tissue and laser osteotomy justify separate discussion.

EFFECTS OF LASERS ON TISSUE

It has been shown in previous chapters that lasers affect tissue in one of three ways: photothermally, photomechanically, and photo-chemically. The most common use for the laser at this time is photothermal; thus, for the most part, lasers used in surgery are effective because of their gross thermal effects on tissues (*i.e.*, they destroy the tissue with concentrated heat). The photothermal effect of lasers varies greatly, however, depending on the following parameters: power density, time of exposure, pulse mode, laser wavelength, and the absorption capacity of the tissue being exposed to the laser energy.

The power density of the laser is equal to the power of the incident laser beam per square centimeter or

$$\text{power density} = \frac{\text{power (watts)}}{\text{area (cm}^2)}$$

Power density is also referred to as *irradience.*

The duration of exposure determines the total energy absorbed by the tissue exposed to the laser. Total energy is measured in joules and is termed *energy density*. Thus,

$$\text{energy density} = \frac{\text{power (watts)} \times \text{time (seconds)}}{\text{area (cm}^2\text{)}}$$

$$\text{or energy density} = \frac{\text{joules}}{\text{cm}^2}$$

The surgeon can manipulate the power density and energy density to control the laser-induced temperature changes in the tissues. It is possible, therefore, to produce three distinct thermal effects on tissue depending on how high the temperature in the tissue is raised by the laser. At temperatures of 35°C to 55°C, tissues are warmed but changes are reversible, so no tissue damage occurs if the elevated temperatures are not maintained. If temperatures are raised to 60°C, denaturation and permanent tissue changes take place. In the 55°C to 60°C range, there is fusion of collagen fibers in connective tissues. This results in "welding," or fusion, of the exposed tissues, a phenomenon that is proving useful in tissue repairs. Between 60°C and 100°C, the tissue is killed by the laser energy but remains in the surgical field. It will slough off gradually over a period of several days. If the temperature of the tissue is raised above 100°C, the water in the tissue boils and vaporizes. The cells explode and disappear in the laser plume, leaving only a rim of charred and carbonized material behind. The low tissue temperatures that result in the welding effect are caused by power densities in the range of 50 watts/cm². These low power densities are only obtainable with milliwatt CO_2 lasers or Nd:YAG lasers set at 2, 3, or 4 watts of incident power. The vaporizing effect of lasers, on the other hand, is the result of much higher power densities. In a CO_2 laser used for cutting purposes, for example, a setting of 40 watts with a beam focused to 0.2 mm will effectively cut through soft tissue like a scalpel owing to the extremely high temperatures generated. The depth of the laser cut varies with the time of exposure; the longer the exposure, the deeper the cut.

Two other parameters that are of critical importance in laser use are the wavelength and absorptive capacity of the tissue exposed to the laser. One of four things can happen to laser energy directed at a surface: It can be transmitted through the surface, it can be reflected, it can be scattered, or it can be absorbed. These phenomena are easily understood if one considers how various substances affect electromagnetic energy in the visible spectrum. Clear glass transmits light, polished metallic surfaces reflect it, white surfaces reflect and scatter it, and black surfaces absorb it. Various lasers at specific wavelengths behave the same way. Because the laser energy affects the tissue only if it is absorbed, the wavelength of the laser and the absorptive capacity of the tissue involved become vital factors in laser usage.

The standard CO_2 laser has a wavelength of 10,600 nm or 10.6 μ in the far infrared spectrum. This wavelength is heavily absorbed in water. Because most tissues contain cells filled with water, the energy of the CO_2 laser is promptly absorbed by the cells, causing them to burst and vaporize. At high power densities, this occurs almost instantaneously, causing little or no effect on the surrounding tissues. The effect of the CO_2 laser, then, is very precise in soft tissue and cartilage; however, bone, which is dense and of low water content, is difficult to cut or vaporize with a CO_2 laser. At high power densities and with prolonged radiant exposure, it is possible to cut bone with a CO_2 laser, but this is less easily accomplished than with a saw or osteotome.

The Nd:YAG laser in common use has a wavelength of 1064 nm or 1.064 μ. Energy at this wavelength, in the near infrared spectrum, is minimally absorbed by water and is thus transmitted by it. The Nd:YAG laser, therefore, can be used in a liquid medium, such as in arthroscopic operations in which a joint is distended with fluid. The Nd:YAG laser, which does not "see" the water, does "see" protein and pigmented substances such as hemoglobin and melanin. Electromagnetic energy in the 1.064-μ wavelength emitted by the Nd:YAG laser is thus absorbed by these materials. The energy of the Nd:YAG laser beam, unlike that of the CO_2 laser beam, is not totally absorbed in the first few cell layers in the tissue in which it is directed. It distributes its heat over a larger area, penetrating deeper into the tissue. The depth of penetration by the incident energy can be as much as 6 mm, and the energy is scattered into the adjoining cell layers. Because the energy of the Nd:YAG laser is distributed over a larger volume of tissue, the heat generated by this device is less than that produced by a CO_2 laser beam. The CO_2 laser has a surface effect, with only minimal penetration caused by the sharply localized release of all the incident energy. The Nd:YAG laser of comparable energy raises the temperature of a larger volume of tissue, but the temperature elevation in the affected tissue is not as great. Raising the power of the incident Nd:YAG laser, however, will not cause deeper penetration of the tissue, but it will raise the temperature of the tissue reached by the energy of the laser beam. The net effect of the Nd:YAG laser is therefore tissue necrosis, and the "cooked" necrotic tissue must slough away after several days. It is possible to obtain a vaporizing effect on pigmented tissue with higher power settings using the Nd:YAG laser, but the deep penetration of the laser beam may damage deeper structures. Because orthopaedic tissues (cartilage and bone) do not absorb energy well in the Nd:YAG spectrum, very high power settings must be used to achieve the desired effect when operating on these tissues with a Nd:YAG laser.

The other parameter of laser use that must be considered is the pulse mode. When a CO_2 laser beam is used for the purpose of precise dissection, the surgeon should select a high power density that is delivered as quickly as possible. This type of usage minimizes the chance of heat being spread to other tissues. This kind of laser surgery can be best performed with the use of the superpulse mode as described in Chapter 2 (Laser Delivery Systems). The superpulse mode and pulse modes used in most medical lasers involve a controlled gating interposed on a continuous beam. The true pulsed lasers have very short (pico- or femtosecond) high-energy bursts that cause a nonlinear effect on the incident tissue. This effect has been called by various names, including photodecomposition, plasma decomposition, and photovaporization. These truly pulsed, or Q-switched, lasers are currently used almost exclusively for ophthalmic or lithotripsy surgery. Tissue ablation performed with a low power density requires longer periods of exposure. In this situation, one should use a continuous gated or pulsed mode of laser energy for preselected fractions of a second.

With this background, the discussion will proceed to a consideration of the effects of the CO_2 and Nd:YAG lasers on bone. Only a limited amount of research has been done on these subjects by a relatively small number of investigators; their work is discussed, and our own observations are briefly presented. Lasers have not been widely adapted to orthopaedics, so what is presented here will probably be superceded relatively soon by newer information. In addition, other types of lasers that are still being developed will probably be adapted more successfully to orthopaedic applications in the future.

EFFECTS OF LASERS ON BONE

It is quicker and easier to cut bone mechanically than with the lasers that are currently available because the density, hardness, and relative lack of moisture of bone make it more reflective of laser energy than soft tissue.[2] In order to penetrate bone with the laser beam, the surgeon is forced to use a high power setting in a focused beam for a long period of time. This is especially true for thick cortical bone. Thin cortical bone and cancellous bone can be cut or penetrated somewhat more easily, but laser techniques are not, for most orthopaedic operations, better or faster than standard mechanical methods.

With the high energy densities needed to cut bone, the surgeon can cause thermal necrosis in adjacent bone tissue.[5,6] The thickness of the rim of necrotic tissue is not likely to be known by the surgeon using a laser to perform an osteotomy, and the consequences of leaving a rim of necrotic bone tissue adjacent to the cut surface may vary. There is relatively little experimental evidence to help settle these points. Tauber and colleagues[12] reported that fracture union in rabbits after osteotomy using the CO_2 laser was slower than in the control animals for the first few weeks postoperatively. At the end of 6 weeks, however, the osteotomies made with the laser were as well healed as the osteotomies made with a saw. Mechanical testing also demonstrated that osteotomies in both groups had similar strengths, as shown by testing of loads to failure at the end of 2 months. Tauber and associates[12] suggested that thermal injury to adjacent bone tissue in the area of the laser osteotomy might have caused initial delay in healing. Small and colleagues[10] however, found that healing of rabbit tibial osteotomies healed more slowly when done with a laser. Despite these concerns, laser osteotomy has found clinical application in otolaryngology. Laser turbinectomy as an adjunct to rhinoplasty was reported by Selkin.[9] Clauser and associates,[3,4] Tang,[11] and Pao-Chang and colleagues[8] also reported on their experimental use of the laser in maxillofacial surgery. Clauser[3,4] and Balin and associates[1] reported that the laser can penetrate thin cortical bone and cancellous bone with acceptably low energy densities without the danger of causing significant thermal necrosis in adjacent bone tissue. They found that a focused beam with a small spot size delivered in a pulse mode significantly diminished damage to adjacent tissues. Balin and colleagues[1] noted that the power required to penetrate the bone was a function of the thickness of the bone; the thicker the bone, the more power was required when the time of exposure was kept constant. They also found that cortical bone required much more energy for penetration of a given thickness than cancellous bone. The energy required for penetration had a linear relationship to the thickness of the bone tissue, and owing to the reflection of the laser from cortical bone, the line defining the energy for penetration – thickness relationship for cortical bone had a much sharper incline than the line defining the same relationship for cancellous bone.

Nuss and colleagues[7] studied the bone ablation characteristics of four infrared lasers: Nd:YAG ($\lambda = 1.064\ \mu$), Hol:YSGG ($\lambda = 2.10\ \mu$), Erb:YAG ($\lambda = 2.94\ \mu$), and CO_2 ($\lambda = 101.6\ \mu$). The evaluations were made on both continuous wave and pulsed modes for the Nd:YAG and CO_2 laser and on pulse lasers in the Nd:YAG, Hol:YSGG, and Erb:YAG types of lasers. These investigators studied the etch rates, histology, and infrared spectrophotometry of bone with each of these lasers. They found that the organic matrix of bone has four major absorption bands in the infrared spectrum at 30.3 μ, 6.06 μ, 6.54 μ, and 8.06 μ. The mineral component of bone absorbs primarily in the 2.94-μ and 9.26-μ bands in the infrared spectrum, and the absorption peak for water and bone is in the 3.0-μ band. They observed that of the four types of laser studied, a pulsed Erb:YAG laser operating in the 2.94-μ band produced the best cutting of bone. The bone was cut with only a 10-μ to 15-μ depth of apparent thermal injury on either side of the area of ablation. They postulated that the Erb:YAG laser ablated bone primarily in a "plasma-cutting" manner with very little thermal component to the ablation mechanism. They suggested that the pulsed Erb:YAG laser created a plasma or ionized state in which electrons are freely dissociated from their atoms. The creation of the plasma state in bone presumably results in bone ablation with almost no thermal injury. These studies were carried out on fresh guinea-pig calvaria. The authors' results are not directly transferable to the clinical situation encountered in orthopaedics because the bone cutting and ablation required in a clinical setting would make much greater demands on the laser. The use of the Erb:YAG laser is also restricted because "at this time there is no optic fiber that offers significant transmissibility and flexibility to be useful."[7]

In our experiments on the effects of lasers on bone, we evaluated the acute effects of laser energy on human bone tissue removed at amputation. Transverse penetration of cadaveric tibial bone was performed on 20 specimens at varying power densities, and these areas were grossly measured and observed. Histologic staining with hematoxylin and eosin was then performed.

Microscopic evaluation showed laser-penetration defects in the bone. The size of the defect depended upon the power density used; at lower power densities, for example, a larger defect developed. This correlates with the increased amount of time required for penetration at these lower power densities. Depending upon the power densities used, sizes of the defects ranged from 0.7 mm to 0.2 mm. With the larger defects, a grey, charred appearance could be noted around the edges of the laser defect. Microscopic evaluation revealed three zones about the laser spot. The first zone was the char zone, which had no discernible structure except a few nondescript particles. The second was a burn zone of variable thickness that had a roughened edge and a carbonaceous-appearing background. The third zone was the osteonecrotic zone, which had intact-appearing bone but empty lacunae, some of which contained pycnotic nuclei (Fig. 5–1).

We also evaluated the response of bone to laser energy in dogs 2,

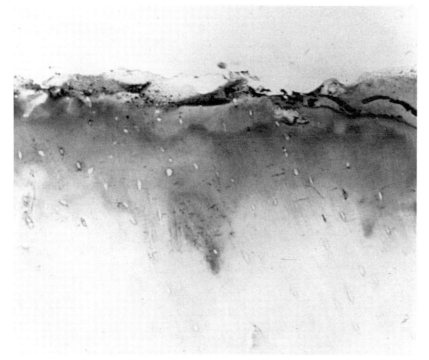

Figure 5–1. Photomicrograph of human cortical bone stained with hematoxylin and eosin. The cut in the tissue has been made in the longitudinal axis of a CO_2 laser osteotomy performed with a continuous-mode 80-watt beam. The char and carbonized deposits are visible on the surface of the bone. There appears to be a change in the staining properties of the tissue for a depth of $250\ \mu$ to $300\ \mu$ beneath the cut surface, and the lacunal of the bone are empty. These changes suggest thermal changes in the bone.

4, and 6 weeks after exposure of the bone to the laser beam. These chronic effects were evaluated with both CO_2 and Nd:YAG lasers. A procedure with transverse laser penetration was performed on the iliac crest of anesthetized adult dogs.

Just prior to surgery, the dogs were given 15 mg/kg of tetracycline intravenously; 1 week prior to harvesting of the iliac bones, they were given 20 mg/kg of oxytetracycline. After removal of the bone, which was penetrated by the laser beam, the effected tissue was studied histologically using decalcified sections stained with hematoxylin and eosin and undecalcified bone stained with trichrome. The tetracycline and oxytetracycline, which were administered preoperatively and 1 week prior to sacrifice, made it possible to evaluate the fluorochrome labeling of osteoid before and after exposure to the laser.

Two weeks after surgery, the bone surrounding the carbonized rim was fragmented and stained poorly with the trichrome (Col. Figs. 5–2 and 5–3). For a distance of 0.5 mm from the center of the

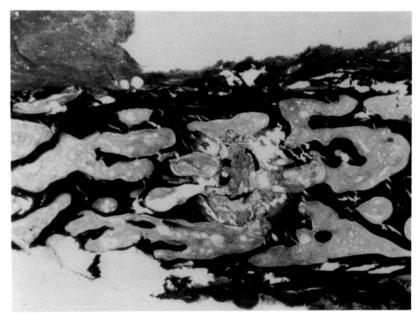

Figure 5–2. Photomicrograph of undecalcified canine cancellous bone stained with trichrome 2 weeks after a CO_2 laser (continuous-mode 50-watt) beam had been used to create a defect in the iliac crest. The bone surrounding the carbonized rim is fragmented and stains poorly with the trichrome. Granulation tissue has begun to fill the laser defect.

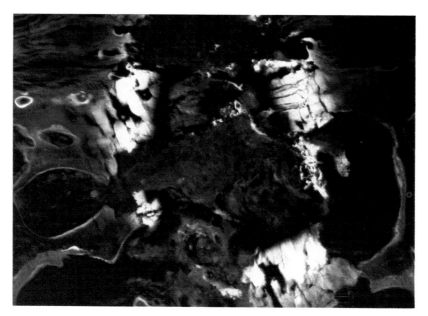

Figure 5–3. Same specimen shown in Figure 5–2, now viewed with fluorescent light. There is extensive fluorochrome labeling of the osteoid bone surrounding the carbonized rim, indicating that the bone tissue about the laser defect had been killed by the heat of the laser. The fluorochrome label is taken up by the open calcium-binding site.

laser defect, there was extensive nondescript fluorochrome labeling with the tetracycline, which had been administered at the time of surgery. This appeared to indicate that the bone tissue about the laser defect had been killed by the heat of the laser beam, because the fluorochrome label is taken up by open calcium binding sites. These bindings sites become randomly arranged with necrosis and denaturation. There was active penetration of this necrotic bone by well-vascularized granulation tissue, however, and the laser defect was filled by the same tissue, which appeared to be depositing new bone with wide osteoid seams labeled by the oxytetracycline. Osteocytes showed variable and decreasing effects from the laser energy as distance increased. The osteocytes identified along the edge of the osteonecrotic zone showed minimal to no effect (Fig. 5–4 and Col. Fig. 5–5).

Our studies have shown that the incident laser beam from both the CO_2 and Nd:YAG lasers causes tissue necrosis in bone in the region immediately adjacent to the laser defect. The necrotic area is

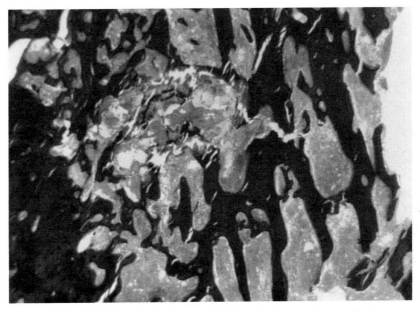

Figure 5–4. Photomicrograph of undecalcified canine tissue stained with trichrome 4 weeks after creation of a transverse defect in the iliac crest with a 50-watt continuous-mode CO_2 laser. The poorly staining necrotic bone tissue about the carbonaceous rim has almost all been removed. The defect is filled with granulation tissue.

variable in width, and its width appeared roughly related to the energy of the incident laser. Wider necrotic areas seemed to be produced by an incident beam set at lower powers. In experimental animals, however, there appeared to be rapid replacement of necrotic bone and prompt filling in of the laser defect.

It is apparent that new lasers and new technologies will have to be utilized in laser osteotomy. The excimer lasers currently under development seem to be the most promising in this regard. Early experiments using bench-model excimer lasers have shown excellent results, producing osteotomies with no thermal necrosis by means of photodecomposition. The lasers available presently for clinical use are much too weak for osteotomies of bone. Newer excimer lasers with fairly large power ranges, stability, and durability are being reported, however.

One final experimental and somewhat controversial use of lasers in surgery on bones is that of stimulating the production of new bone. Several reports indicate that milliwatt CO_2 lasers and low-

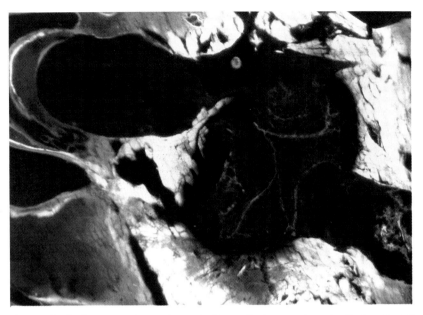

Figure 5–5. Same specimen shown in Figure 5–4, now viewed with fluorescent light. Wide seams of osteoid that are labeled green by oxytetracycline, which was administered 1 week prior to sacrifice, are apparent, indicating rapid formation of new bone about the laser spot.

power Nd:YAG lasers may stimulate new bone formation in rabbit calvarial defect models. The use of lasers in the visible spectrum for the same purpose has been described in several reports, and the effectiveness of the so-called cold lasers remains under investigation. This topic is considered in Chapter 12 (Cold Lasers).

REFERENCES

1. Balin PL, Wheeland AG: Carbon dioxide laser perforation of exposed cranial bone to stimulate granulation tissue. Plas Reconstr Surg 75:898–902, 1985
2. Biyikli S, Modest MF: Energy requirements for osteotomy of femora and tibiae with a moving CW CO_2 laser. Lasers Surg Med 7:512–519, 1987
3. Clauser C: Comparison of depth and profile of osteotomies performed

by rapid superpulsed and continuous wave CO_2 laser beams at high power output. J Oral Maxillofac Surg 44:425–430, 1986

4. Clauser C, Panzoni E: Comparison between rapid superpulsed and continuous CO_2 laser for osteotomies. In Atsumi K, Nimschel K (eds): Laser Tokyo '81, pp 4–6. Japan, Inter Group Corp., 1981

5. Clayman, L, Fuller TA, Beckman H: Healing of continuous wave and rapid superpulsed carbon dioxide laser-induced bone defects. J Oral Surg 36:932–937, 1978

6. Gertzbein SD, DeDemeter D, Cruickshank B et al: The effect of laser osteotomy on bone healing. Lasers Surg Med 1:361–373, 1981

7. Nuss RC, Fabian RL, Sorker R et al: Infrared laser bone ablation. Lasers Surg Med 8:381–391, 1988

8. Pao-Chang M, Xiou-X, Hin Z et al: Preliminary report on the application of the CO_2 laser scalpel for operations on the maxillofacial bones. Lasers Surg Med 1:375–384, 1981

9. Selkin SG: Laser turbinectomy as an adjunct to rhinoseptoplasty. Arch Otolaryngol 11:446–449, 1985

10. Small IA, Osborn TP, Fuller TA et al: Observations of carbon dioxide laser and bone burr in the osteotomy of the rabbit tibia. J Oral Surg 37:159, 1979

11. Tang XM: Effect of CO_2 laser irradiation on experimental fracture healing: A transmission electron microscope study. Lasers Surg Med 6:346–352, 1986

12. Tauber C, Farine I, Horoszowski H et al: Fracture healing in rabbits after osteotomy using the CO_2 laser. Acta Orthop Scand 50:385–390, 1979

6

Lower Extremity Amputation with the CO$_2$ Laser*

John V. White
John D. Cunningham

Although simple in concept, performance of an amputation of the lower extremity can be a complex task for the surgeon. Patients requiring these procedures are often debilitated from multisystem disease. More than half of patients requiring amputation for severe ischemia have diabetes and severe cardiopulmonary disease, including angina, chronic congestive heart failure, and chronic obstructive lung disease.[1] The requirement for amputations in this population is most frequently endstage ischemia manifesting with distal gangrene, nonhealing ulcers or wounds, or severe pain at rest. Infection of ischemic tissue and edema are frequent accompaniments. Preoperative preparation of the patient to improve cardiopulmonary status and reduce distal edema and infection is frequently limited by the severity of distal tissue loss. Understandably, then, the operative mortality of lower-extremity amputation is high, ranging from 6% to 30%.[2,3] Major causes of mortality include cardiac and respiratory complications and progressive infection with sepsis.[4] Those patients who tolerate amputation also face a high morbidity. A recent analysis of amputations in peripheral vascular occlusive disease documented delays in healing due to stump infection in 27.6% of patients.[5] The organisms cultured from these infected stumps included *Pseudomonas, Staphylococcus aureus, Klebsiella, Enterobacter*, and other organisms most frequently cultured from ischemic foot infections. Recent experimental evidence has suggested that distal-soft-tissue infections may seed lymphatics.[6] Transection of the lym-

*This work was supported by NHLBI grant HL34104-02.

phatics at the surgical site permits lymph leakage and bacterial deposition within the sterile field. Such contamination may account for the subsequent infection.[7]

Some authors have recommended the performance of staged amputations to eliminate seeding of the amputation stump. McIntyre[8] has suggested that guillotine amputation of the foot followed by delayed performance of below- or above-knee amputations can decrease the infectious complications of one-stage amputation; however, this approach requires subjecting often severely debilitated patients to a minimum of two surgical procedures.

Because of our desire to limit the potential for bacterial contamination of the surgical wound, we began to explore the use of the CO_2 laser for the performance of lower-extremity amputations.

The CO_2 laser has a wavelength of 10.6 nm, which is in the mid-infrared portion of the spectrum. The invisible beam is mirror directed and targeted with a coaxial helium–neon laser. Energy from the CO_2 laser interacts with tissue through a photothermal process. On contact with cells, the light energy is converted to heat and intracellular water is instantly vaporized, causing cellular disruption. Because water absorbs and dissipates CO_2 laser energy, vital tissues can easily be protected with saline-moistened towels and pads.

The CO_2 laser has a number of special characteristics that are useful for soft tissue dissection. Its noncontact method of tissue division permits minimal tissue handling, which minimizes tissue injury. In addition, less manipulation of the soft tissues forces less lymph and bacteria through the transected lymphatics. Another major advantage of the CO_2 laser is its ability to seal lymphatics and small blood vessels as it transects tissues, once again minimizing the deposition of distal bacteria into the surgical field. Because the CO_2 laser beam has a temperature of 1500°C, it seals small lymphatics and blood vessels with heat and sterilizes tissues as it divides. For these reasons, we have used this laser to perform both minor and major amputations of the lower extremity for the past 3 years.

TECHNIQUE

Once the need for amputation is established, the patient is appropriately prepared for surgery. Fluid status, electrolyte levels, blood sugar, and blood pH are regulated. Cardiopulmonary status and renal status are optimized. Control of infection is attempted with intravenous administration of bacteria-specific antibiotics for 48 to 72 hours prior to surgery if possible. Edema of the extremity is reduced with elevation during this time.

Patients are evaluated both clinically and in the vascular laboratory to determine the appropriate level of amputation. Clinically, skin viability and integrity, and the absence of adjacent soft-tissue infection and draining wounds are determined. Segmental arterial Doppler studies and pulse-volume recordings of the high and low thigh, calf, and ankle are obtained. Pressures greater than 60 mm Hg with pulsatile flow documented by pulse-volume recordings at a given level suggest that the likelihood of healing an amputation at that location is greater than 90%.[9] When preoperative preparation of the patient is completed, surgical consent for amputation with CO_2 laser is obtained.

Once in the operating room, the patient is placed in the supine position upon the operating table. General or regional anesthesia is utilized to anesthetize the extremity so that the patient is comfortable and an absolutely stable field can be created. The skin is washed with Betadine soap scrub and then prepped with Betadine solution, which is allowed to dry. Standard disposable surgical drapes are used to establish the sterile field (Fig. 6–1). Plastic drapes or

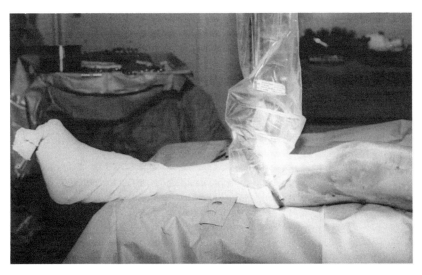

Figure 6–1. Sterile draping of the surgical field, and proper adjustment of the articulating arm of the CO_2 laser.

stockinettes on the extremity are specifically avoided to prevent melting of this material by the laser. Saline-soaked sterile towels are wrapped around the leg just above and below the lines of surgical incision to protect the tissues (Fig. 6–2).

When the sterile field has been created, the laser is moved into position, the articulated arm is dressed with a sterile laser drape, and the 125-mm handpiece is connected to the lens. The articulating arm is adjusted with column height and counterbalance weights so that the handpiece floats just above the area of leg to be incised (Fig. 6–3). All members of the operating team and the patient must be wearing laser safety glasses with clear plastic lenses prior to turning on the laser.

Laser function is confirmed at a power setting of 30 watts, mode of single impulse, and a pulse duration of 0.1 seconds. A single impulse in focused and a second in defocused mode are made on a tongue blade (see Fig. 6–3). The tongue blade is examined to confirm an appropriate penetration with the focused spot and a superficial effect of the defocused spot.

For division of tissue, 20 watts is used for patients with thin,

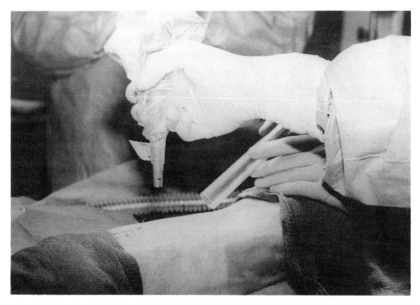

Figure 6–2. Protection of vital tissues from CO_2 laser energy with saline-soaked towels.

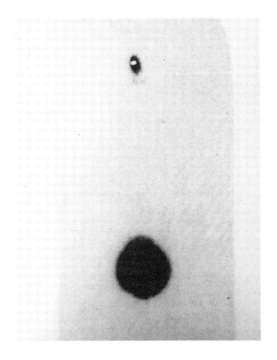

Figure 6-3. Tongue blade confirming appropriate laser function at a power of 30 watts. Focused beam (*top*) cleanly penetrates wood and defocused beam (*bottom*) produces a superficial char.

somewhat atrophic extremities, and 40 watts is used for those patients with thick, edematous extremities. The first assistant holds the smoke evacuator approximately 2 cm from the area of laser-tissue contact. With his other hand, he places countertraction opposite to the surgeon (Fig. 6-4). The incision for the anterior flap is made from the skin down through subcutaneous tissue until the bone is clearly exposed. A small flash of flame indicates complete division of the periosteum and etching of the bone, itself. Care is taken during this process to maintain the laser beam at an angle that will contact only the tissue to be divided. The angle should be chosen so that once this tissue is divided, the only other structure the laser could contact would be a wet towel. After the anterior surface of the leg is divided, the leg is rotated slightly medially and laterally to enable division of the posterior flap and muscle (Fig. 6-5). The major neurovascular bundles are isolated, clamped, divided, and separately tied. No attempt is made to coagulate these structures with the laser. Once all soft tissue and muscle have been completely divided and the bone circumferentially exposed, the periosteum is raised proximally for a distance of 1 cm above the anterior flap with

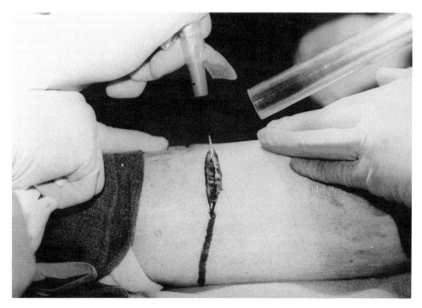

Figure 6-4. Gentle countertraction of tissues by surgeon and assistant. Note proximity of smoke evacuator.

a periosteal elevator. A Gigli saw is used to transect bone. Because bone is anhydrous, it divides very slowly under even high-power CO_2 laser energy. The bone division is therefore performed in standard fashion. The specimen is passed from the field when transection is complete. There is usually very little bleeding at the completion of the laser amputation because the laser seals small blood vessels and lymphatics. Those areas of persistent bleeding are clamped and ligated with a fine absorbable suture. Bleeding marrow is controlled with wax. The stump is irrigated copiously with normal saline solution to completely remove bone particles. Closure is accomplished in standard fashion with the muscles of the posterior flap being fixed to the anterior periosteum to provide an appropriate pad. Subcutaneous tissues are reapproximated with absorbable sutures, and the skin is closed with interrupted simple and mattress sutures of 3-0 and 4-0 nylon. A sterile dressing is applied. Rigid dressings are placed where appropriate.

Standard postoperative care is employed. The wound is carefully evaluated on a daily basis and sutures are left in until there is clear evidence of healing. Despite the use of laser, healing averages 18 to 21 days.

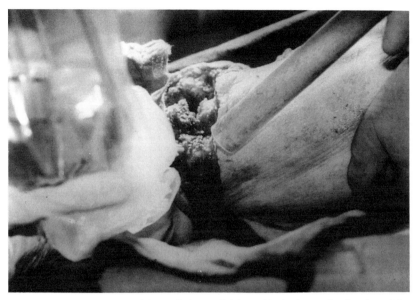

Figure 6-5. Completion of the soft-tissue division with the laser. Application of the defocused mode of laser energy is used to coagulate small blood vessels prior to their transection.

RESULTS

This technique has been used for major and minor amputations in more than 18 patients. All amputations were accomplished at the level chosen preoperatively. No technical difficulties were encountered. Tissue division with the laser was performed cleanly in a completely noncontact fashion. No injury due to uncontrolled laser energy occurred to the patient or the surgical team. Operative time and blood loss for amputations performed with the CO_2 laser were similar to those recorded for standard amputations.

Healing proceeded normally. Occasional suture-track infections were noted, but no deep-space infections developed. All patients with suitable strength and coordination were fitted with prostheses. The laser-amputated stump accepted weight bearing without problem (Fig. 6-6A and B).

Less stump edema was observed during convalescence of these patients. This may result from preoperative preparation of the patient, less tissue instrumentation and manipulation, and the sealing of lymphatics by the laser. Coincident with this observation was the report by patients of less postoperative discomfort. Although this benefit of CO_2-laser amputation is difficult to substantiate, it may stem from the reduction in edema, especially in the perineural tissues.

CONCLUSIONS

The CO_2 laser provides a significant advantage to the performance of lower-extremity amputation. Its noncontact method of tissue division produces less tissue trauma and manipulation than electrocautery. The photothermal process sterilizes as it cuts. These benefits of laser use can serve to reduce directly the greatest causes of morbidity of patients undergoing amputation. Sensibly applied, the CO_2 laser can enhance the surgeon's ability to deal more effectively with the complex and challenging problem of lower-extremity amputation.

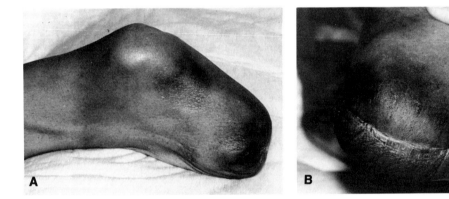

Figure 6–6. *A* and *B*, Appearance of below-knee amputation stump (amputation performed with CO_2 laser) after 6 months of weight bearing on a standard prosthesis.

REFERENCES

1. Castronuovo JJ, Deane LM, Deterling RA et al: Below-knee amputation. Arch Surg 115:1184–1187, 1980
2. Porter JM, Baur GM, Taylor LM Jr: Lower-extremity amputations for ischemia. Arch Surg 116:89–92, 1981
3. Otteman MG, Stahlgren LH: Evaluation of factors which influence mortality and morbidity following major lower extremity amputation for arteriosclerosis. Surg Gynecol Obstet 120:1217–1220, 1965
4. Keagy BA, Schwartz JA, Kotb M et al: Lower extremity amputation: The control series. J Vasc Surg 4:321–326, 1986
5. Berardi RS, Keonin Y: Amputations in peripheral vascular occlusive disease. Am J Surg 135:231–234, 1978
6. Rubin JR, Malone JM, Goldstone J: The role of the lymphatic system in acute arterial prosthetic graft infections. J Vasc Surg 2:92–97, 1985
7. White JV, Freda J, Kozar R et al: Does bacteremia pose a direct threat to synthetic vascular grafts? Surgery 102:402–408, 1987
8. McIntyre KE, Bailey SA, Malone JM et al: Guillotine amputation in the treatment of nonsalvageable lower extremity infections. Arch Surg 119:450–453, 1984
9. Moore WS: Amputation level determination. In Rutherford R (ed): Vascular Surgery. Philadelphia, WB Saunders Co, 1984

7

Revision Arthroplasty Using a CO$_2$ Laser

Henry H. Sherk
Charles Kollmer

THE EXPERIMENTAL BASIS OF REMOVAL OF BONE CEMENT

Over the past several years, the number of patients requiring revision surgery with removal of polymethylmethacrylate (PMMA) after failed total hip arthroplasty has progressively increased, and the number can be expected to increase further. The surgical method presently used for removing bone cement in revision arthroplasty is mechanical and requires the use of high-speed burrs, reamers, and other instruments that often cause fractures or bone penetration, thus prolonging or complicating patient recovery (Fig. 7–1). A safe, efficient, and effective alternative method of removing PMMA would be of benefit to patients required to undergo revision arthroplasty.

The first reports of the use of the CO$_2$ laser to remove bone cement in revision arthroplasty appeared approximately 10 years ago.[1] The concentrated heat of the CO$_2$ laser in transforming PMMA almost instantaneously from a solid to gaseous form provided the basis of interest in the use of the laser for this purpose. Before using the laser clinically, however, it seemed important to us to evaluate the following: heat transfer from PMMA to bone during laser use, comparative absorptive capacities of laser energy at λ 10,600 nm — bone versus PMMA, gaseous products of vaporization of PMMA, and histologic changes in bone after removal of PMMA with a laser.

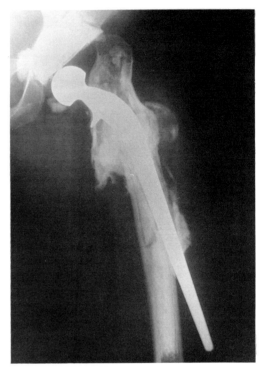

Figure 7-1. Anteroposterior roentgenogram of a failed total-hip revision carried out by conventional techniques. The hip is dislocated, the femoral shaft has been fractured, and the long-stemmed prosthesis has been directed out through a fenestration in the shaft into the soft tissues. Damage to the femoral shaft by high-speed reamers is a constant problem in surgery for total-hip revision.

Heat Transfer from PMMA to Bone During Laser Use

The CO_2 laser removes PMMA by means of a photothermal reaction. The PMMA is virtually instantaneously heated to a level beyond its vaporization temperature and converted to a gaseous substance. Because the laser beam is not uniformly powerful throughout the laser spot, however, there are probably areas within the spot in which the temperature rises, but not high enough to cause vaporization (Fig. 7-2A and B). This is especially true if the beam is defocused or directed obliquely onto the working surface (Fig. 7-2C). Under these circumstances, there will be areas in the laser spot in which the energy of the laser will remain in the PMMA as heat. When this occurs, the temperature might rise high enough to produce thermal injury to the adjacent bone.

We decided to measure these temperatures directly. We secured

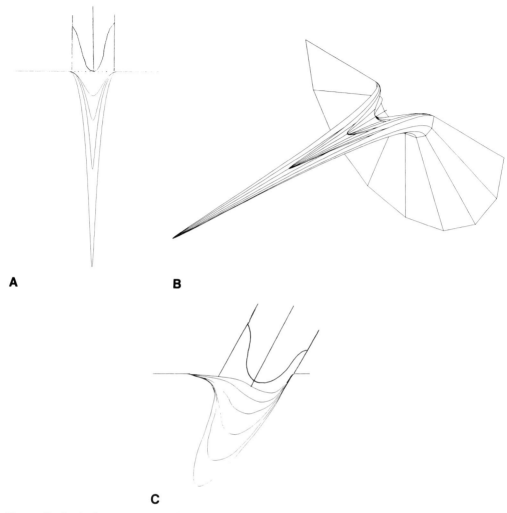

Figure 7–2. *A*, Cut profile for a CO$_2$ laser in soft tissue by a gaussian beam normal to the tissue surface. Each successive curve represents the tissue surface at progressive increments of time. The aspect ratio (i.e., length:width) increases owing to the concentration of the beam at the apex by oblique reflection off the steep crater walls. This gaussian configuration results in a concentration of laser power in the center of the spot. At the margins of the spot, power is lower, and the temperature in this area may not be high enough to produce instantaneous vaporization of the PMMA. The heat of the laser can therefore be absorbed by the PMMA and cause the local temperature to rise. *B*, 3-dimensional diagram of *A*. *C*, Cut profile for a CO$_2$ laser in soft tissue by a gaussian beam not normal to the tissue surface. Each successive curve is now wider than for the normal case, with a slight convexity to the upper surface due to reflection of the beam off the lower surface. There is a larger area in the laser spot in which the temperature is not high enough to vaporize the PMMA; therefore, the temperature of the PMMA is likely to rise more quickly.

thermocouples (Alpha Engineering Company) to the outer cortex of a 4-inch long midshaft segment of a cadaveric femur. We drilled 1.5-mm holes of varying depths into the bony cortex. The cortex and medullary canal were instrumented with additional thermocouples. With the specimen placed in a 37°C bath, we implanted Simplex bone cement into the medullary canal of the femoral shaft fragment. Temperatures were recorded during the setting of PMMA at the cement core, at the bone–cement interface, midcortex, and on the surface of the bone (Fig. 7–3). Core temperatures of 80°C were obtained, with cement–bone interface temperatures of 55°C and midcortical temperatures ranging downward to 40°C on the surface of the bone. We then removed the PMMA with a CO_2 laser using a waveguide (Heraus Laser Sonics) set at 20 watts in a continuous-wave mode (Fig. 7–4A and B). During vaporization of the PMMA, we recorded two separate temperature values at the bone–cement interface—the absolute maximum and the sustained maximum. The absolute maximum lasted less than 1 second and appeared to represent the direct exposure of the area overlying the thermocouple to the laser beam. The sustained maximum represented the temperature peak, which lasted at least 5 seconds. We obtained values of 55°C to 60°C for the absolute maximum and 48°C to 49°C for the sustained maximum. The temperature at the surface of the bone did not exceed 39°C during laser removal of the PMMA (Fig. 7–5).

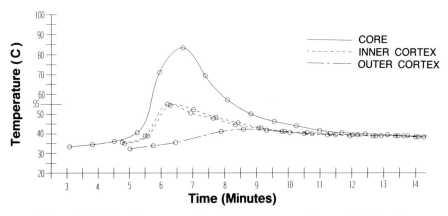

Figure 7–3. Graphic representation of setting temperatures of PMMA at the core, inner cortex, and outer cortex.

It appeared, therefore, that the temperature of the bone–cement interface and the temperature in the cortex of the bone were not higher than those observed during implantation of PMMA. Although the thermal effects of lasing are not known, the thermal effects of implanting PMMA to bone have been extensively investigated. Other authors have shown that setting PMMA generates temperatures up to 100°C in the core of the cement and that temperatures at the bone–cement interface are in the 48°C to 70°C range during setting. These temperatures vary with the ambient temperature in the room, the relative amounts of polymer and monomer, and the time lapse between mixing and implantation. Because proteins denature at the upper limits of the 48°C to 70°C range, the setting PMMA probably causes at least some thermal necrosis of the bone tissue at the bone–cement interface.[7,8,11,14] In actual clinical practice, the thermal effect of the setting PMMA on bone is probably much less significant than the reaming of the bone[4] and the release of free oxygen radicals during setting.[5,10] These mechanical and chemical effects probably destroy more bone tissue than the thermal effects alone; therefore, if an orthopaedic surgeon is willing to accept the mechanical, thermal, and chemical damage to the underlying bone in implantation of PMMA, it seems reasonable to accept the more limited thermal injury caused by removing it with a CO₂ laser.

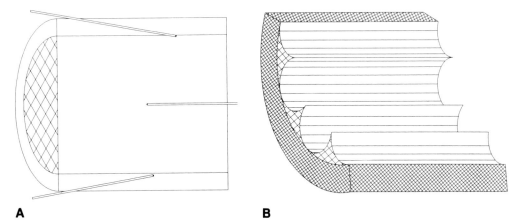

A   **B**

Figure 7–4. *A*, Diagram of placement of thermocouples in the core of the PMMA and in the cortex of the bone. *B*, Diagram of wave guide to remove PMMA. The laser is directed tangential to the endosteal surface of the bone.

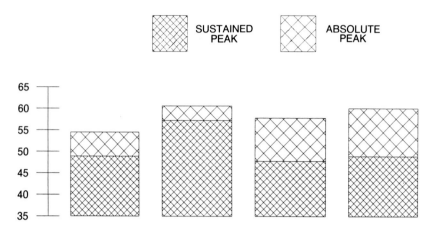

Figure 7-5. Bar graph showing bone temperature during vaporization of PMMA.

Comparative Absorptive Capacities of CO₂ Laser Energy at λ 10,600 nm — Bone versus PMMA

The thermal conductivity, specific heat, density, heat-generation parameters, and infrared spectrophotometry of PMMA and bone have been described in previous reports.[13] Polymethylmethacrylate readily absorbs laser energy in the far infrared spectrum, whereas bone does not. PMMA is thus largely vaporized by the laser, although some of the laser's energy may be retained as heat. The thermal conductivity of PMMA is about half that of bone (0.17 joules per meter, per second, per degree centigrade [Jms°C] for PMMA and 0.29 Jms°C for bone)[8,11,12] so that the heat generated by lasering PMMA is dissipated more slowly through PMMA than through bone. This relative insulating effect of PMMA may offer some protection to bone when PMMA is being vaporized. When bone is subjected to prolonged CO₂ laser exposure, some of the energy is reflected, while some is retained as heat, and because of bone's higher conductivity, the heat is transmitted much more rapidly through bone than through PMMA. If temperatures were to rise above 60°C in the bone, there would be rapid conduction of heat to a wide volume of tissue with real potential for producing extensive thermal injury. It seemed appropriate, therefore, to find the least amount of laser energy required to remove PMMA, with the expectation that this limited degree of power would have less impact on the bone.

To determine the differential responses of PMMA in bone, we prepared plates of PMMA ranging in thickness from 0.5 cm to 1 cm. The thickness of each plate was measured with a caliper. A CO_2 laser beam from a Sharplan 1100 laser focused to a spot size of 0.1 mm was directed transversely at right angles to the plates. Power settings of 10, 15, 20, 30, and 35 watts were utilized in a superpulse mode. The times of penetration of the plates with these power settings and modes were recorded. Thirty to fifty measurements for each plate thickness and power setting were obtained. The same experiment was repeated on segments of fresh human tibial cortical bone removed at amputation. Segments of bone 0.5-cm to 0.9-cm thick were utilized.

We found that laser penetration occurred at least two to ten times more rapidly through PMMA than through bone; in some instances, it occurred 20 times as rapidly ($P < 0.01$). The data were subjected to a three-way ANOVA in which the three factors were substance (PMMA versus bone), thickness (5 mm, 7.5 mm, and 10 mm), and power (15 watts versus 35 watts). Mean penetration times for PMMA did not exceed 1.1 seconds for any thickness. The standard deviations were small (all < 0.12), indicating little variation in the time required for laser penetration.

Mean times for laser penetration of bone consistently exceeded 29 seconds at 15 watts. In only one sample, which was 5-mm thick, did penetration take as little as 25.43 seconds. The times required for penetration of all three thicknesses of bone differed significantly from those with the corresponding PMMA thickness ($P < 0.01$ by unpaired T tests) and differed from each other (Game's and Howell's modification of the Tukey analysis for unequal variances). Variability and standard error were low. The data are shown in Table 7-1. Figures 7-6 and 7-7 demonstrate how the greater time differential for penetration of bone and PMMA occurs at the lower power densities.

We concluded that a low power density of 15 watts to 20 watts removed PMMA completely and effectively. This degree of laser power was reflected by bone, which seemed relatively impervious to it. It was thought that the relatively low power setting of 20 watts in the superpulse or continuous mode should be effective against the PMMA but would not penetrate or injure bone except for the possibility of a superficial thermal injury of a few microns in depth. We noted also that the 20-watt laser produced an orange glow in the substance of the PMMA while vaporization of the bone cement was in progress. When this degree of laser energy struck the cortical

Table 7–1
Relative Penetration Times of PMMA versus Bone by a CO_2 Laser*

	Plate Thickness	Mean Time (Sec)	Standard Deviation
PMMA	5.0 mm		
	15 watts (SP)	0.58	0.04
	35 watts (SP)	0.31	0.06
	7.5 mm		
	15 watts (SP)	0.78	0.12
	35 watts (SP)	0.48	0.03
	10.0 mm		
	15 watts (SP)	1.06	0.09
	35 watts (SP)	0.52	0.07
Bone	5.0 mm		
	15 watts (SP)	29.30	1.04
	35 watts (SP)	0.88	0.08
	7.5 mm		
	15 watts (SP)	81.49	8.97
	35 watts (SP)	1.46	0.18
	10.0 mm		
	15 watts	163.68	18.73
	35 watts (SP)	2.75	0.21

* Varying thicknesses of PMMA and bone were penetrated by the laser at varying power settings. A superpulsed (SP) mode was used for all tests. Thirty to fifty tests were performed for each time measurement. The data obtained for the power settings of 15 watts and 35 watts in the SP mode are shown.

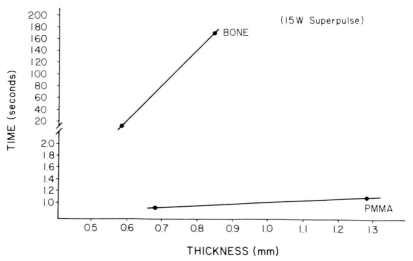

Figure 7–6. Representation of penetration times of varying thicknesses of PMMA and bone by a well-focused CO_2 laser beam set at 35 watts in a superpulse mode. The graph shows bone's resistance to penetration compared to PMMA.

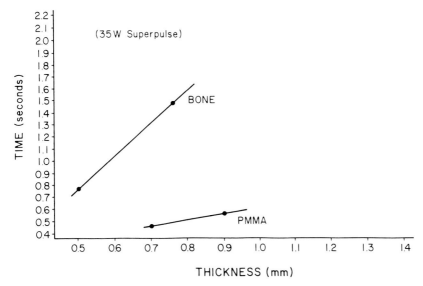

Figure 7-7. Graphic representation of comparative penetration times of bone versus PMMA with a CO_2 laser beam set at 15 watts in a superpulse mode. At this power setting, PMMA is still penetrated very rapidly, but bone penetration by the laser takes up to 20 times as long.

bone, however, a white flash was noted almost instantaneously. The change in the color of the laser directed onto bone versus PMMA appears to serve as a valuable cue that the laser beam has left PMMA and is now directed onto a bony surface. This cue should make it possible to remove the laser beam almost immediately from the bony surface to avoid the possibility of thermal injury.

Gaseous Products of Vaporization of PMMA

Removal of PMMA with a CO_2 laser in revision arthroplasty causes the release of gaseous and particulate material into the operating-room air (Table 7-2). Concerns have arisen regarding the nature of these products and whether they have potential for injury to both the patient and the operating-room staff. In 1983, Horoszowski and colleagues[6] reported that they found an average of 30 ppm of carbon monoxide, 6.4 ppm of formaldehyde, and 1 ppm of hydrogen cyanide in 20 total joint revisions. They found that the products of vaporization of PMMA caused nausea and headaches in the operating-room team when high-power vacuum exhaust systems were not used to

Table 7-2

Gas Chromatography of On-site Flame-ionization of Simplex Bone Cement

Chemical Found	Amount	Threshold Limit
Acrylamide	3 mg/mm³	0.3 mg/mm³
Formaldehyde	12 ppm	1 ppm
Formalin	6 ppm	1 ppm
Hydrocyanic acid	4 ppm	10 ppm
Methane	8 ppm	Asphyxiant at any concentration
Hexane	10 ppm	50 ppm

remove these substances from the room during the phase of the procedure in which the laser was in use.

In 1984, Kroll and colleagues[9] reported that their analysis of vaporization products during laser removal of bone cement yielded methanol, formic acid, formaldehyde, methyl formate, water vapor, acrolein, and acrylic acid. Both Horoszowski and Kroll and their associates commented on the flammability of the gaseous vaporization products of laser removal of PMMA. Horoszowski suggested that a defocused beam directed against dry PMMA had the potential to permit the laser plume to ignite. The defocused beam diffuses more heat into the surrounding PMMA, and it can raise the temperature high enough to ignite the laser plume when flammable substances such as methane and acetylene are present. Kroll suggested the possible need for respiratory isolation in case of a methacrylate fire.

In 1987, Choy and colleagues[3] evaluated the vaporization products of PMMA exposed to an Nd:YAG laser. They found that carbon monoxide comprised 33% and hydrogen comprised 30% of the total. Methane, acetylene, CO_2, and unsaturated hydrocarbons each comprised about 8.5% of the total products of vaporization, and methyl methacrylate, benzene, and other hydrocarbons made up the rest.

In 1987, Booth and colleagues[2] reported that normal constituents of PMMA were detected in the gaseous material collected from PMMA vaporization with a CO_2 laser; in addition, they noted a small amount of formaldehyde (3 ppm). They indicated that Palacos and Simplex yield different amounts of particulate matter (1650 mg/mm³ versus 2250 mg/mm³, respectively).

In our own studies, we secured a number of air-borne samples of the smoke recovered from vaporizing freshly made Simplex bone cement. Using on-site flame-ionization gas chromatography, we identified the substances shown in Table 7–3.

In another study, we evaluated the products of vaporization in the operating room during laser use when PMMA was being removed. In this study, a high-powered vacuum was placed at the edge of the wound so that all visible smoke was immediately sucked away from the operative field into the vacuum filters. Another vacuum tube was placed at the surgeon's shoulder and activated whenever PMMA vaporization was being performed. In two cases, we could detect only an average of 8.6 ppm of unidentifiable hydrocarbons at the surgeon's shoulder. It is reasonable to assume that the concentration of these substances is significantly less elsewhere in the room. These levels are well below the OSHA safety standards of 55 ppm of

Table 7–3
Gaseous Products of Vaporization of PMMA*

Horoszowski M et al[6]

Carbon monoxide	30	ppm
Formaldehyde	6.4	ppm
Hydrogen cyanide	1	ppm

Kroll DA et al[9]

Methanol	Acrolein
Formic acid	Acrylic acid
Formaldehyde	Methyl formate

Choy DSJ et al[3]

Methyl methacrylate	0.22%
Methane	8.8%
Acetylene	8.7%
Unsaturated hydrocarbons	9.35%
Benzene	0.45%
Carbon dioxide	0.035%
Carbon monoxide	33.3%
Hydrogen	30.6%

Medical College of Pennsylvania (1988)

Acrylamide	3 mg/mm³
Formaldehyde	18 ppm
Hydrocyanic acid	4 ppm
Methane	8 ppm
Hexane	10 ppm

* Gaseous products of CO_2 laser vaporization of PMMA as determined by four groups of investigators. The variations in results may represent differences in the origin, age, laser power, temperature, or in vivo versus in vitro testing.

unidentifiable hydrocarbons in the workplace. With the vacuum system in place and functioning during PMMA laser vaporization, it is difficult to detect any odor. The human nose can usually detect substances in air in concentrations of about 50 ppm. It appears, therefore, that the use of the vacuum during surgery removes the harmful products of vaporization and that this is a safe procedure if appropriate precautions are observed (Fig. 7–8).

Inadvertent ignition of the laser plume can be avoided during the use of a free-beam CO_2 laser by keeping the power density at an effective level and by not allowing the tissues to dry. Frequent use of saline mist spray onto the PMMA achieves satisfactory moistening. Ignition of the laser plume is not an issue with the use of a waveguide because the laser fiber incorporates a tube through which a jet of CO_2 is directed onto the working surface. The CO_2 does not support the ignition of the laser plume and prevents the sudden flame-out that is occasionally seen during the use of the free-beam CO_2 laser.[6,9]

The conflicting data and varying results gathered by the aforementioned investigators indicate that further study is required. For

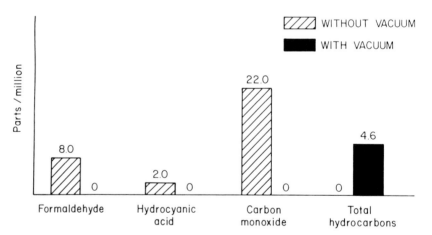

Figure 7–8. Bar graph showing analysis of gaseous products of vaporization during surgery in which a high-powered vacuum system was or was not used. Horoszowski and colleagues[6] found formaldehyde, hydrocyanic acid, and carbon monoxide. When the laser plume was evacuated with the vacuum system in one of our cases, only 4.6 ppm of unidentifiable hydrocarbons were detected in the room. This level is well within the OSHA limit of 55 ppm.

example, freshly made PMMA may yield different products of vaporization than PMMA that has been in the body for many years. In addition, in the clinical situation, products of PMMA vaporization may combine with products of vaporization of blood and other tissues to produce substances quite different from those obtained in the in vitro experiments. Furthermore, the power of the laser and the heat generated may affect what products are obtained. Although these questions remain unanswered, it does appear that the clinical use of the laser to remove PMMA is safe if a high-powered vacuum is used and the gaseous products of vaporization are not permitted to diffuse into the operating-room air.

Histologic Evaluation of Bone after Removal of PMMA with a CO₂ Laser

It is well known that laser energy in the 10,600-nm band does not readily cut bone in the manner required by orthopaedic surgeons. It is possible to divide thinner bones such as the turbinates or nasal septae with little difficulty, but cutting thick cortical bone requires very large amounts of laser energy. Much of this energy is absorbed as heat, and extensive thermal necrosis of bone is thought to occur as a result.[13] To evaluate this phenomenon, we performed an osteotomy of a fresh cadaveric tibia. The osteotomy required 17.6 minutes. The laser handpiece was directed at right angles to the bone. The laser was focused to the smallest spot size possible and set at 15 watts in a superpulse mode. We then decalcified the bone, and after routine preparation of the slides, we reviewed sections of the osteotomy site stained with hematoxylin and eosin. A thin char zone was evident at the surface of the cut bone, and there were changes noted in the staining properties of the bone to a depth of 250μ. The lacunae of the osteocytes that were adjacent to the osteotomy site appeared empty, possibly as a result of thermal denaturation of the cellular proteins. It is apparent that the CO₂ laser will cause significant injury to the cortical bone if used in this way (see Chapt. 5).

We then took 4-inch segments of fresh cadaveric tibiae and filled them with bone cement. We removed the PMMA with a CO₂ laser set at 20 watts that was directed tangential to the bone. The laser was not directed at right angles to the tibial cortex because the procedure of cement removal requires tangential application of the laser energy along the inner aspect of the cortical bone. The full effects of the laser, therefore, were not directed against the bone, such as

87

occurred with the osteotomy. Specimens were removed from the tibia after removal of the cement, and histologic evaluation was carried out after decalcification and staining with hematoxylin and eosin.

On gross inspection of the endosteal surface after cement removal with the laser, there were several patchy areas of darkened bone. Histologically, osteonecrosis was noted in those locations, with the depth of involvement measuring 0.1 mm to 0.7 mm. The remainder of the bone revealed no definite evidence of thermal necrosis and very little change in the staining qualities of the bone beneath the endosteal surface. There was little apparent change in the appearance of the osteocytes in the lacunae beneath the endosteal surface. It appeared, histologically at least, that the tangential application of laser energy produced minimal damage to the bone during cement removal (Fig. 7-9).

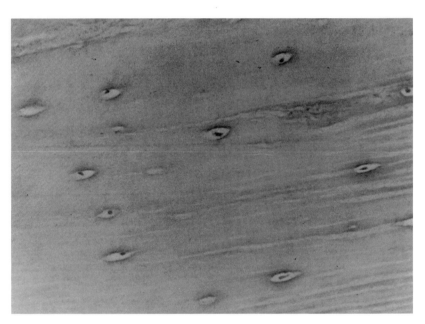

Figure 7-9. Photomicrograph of fresh human tibial cortical bone after vaporization of PMMA with a CO_2 laser from the medullary canal. A small amount of PMMA and the endosteal surface (*upper left*) remains visible. There is no evidence of thermal necrosis of the bone following tangential application of the laser beam. (Original magnification times 100.)

CLINICAL STUDIES: REMOVAL OF PMMA AND REVISION ARTHROPLASTY

To date, we have used CO$_2$ lasers in 38 joint revisions. Initially, the laser seemed to offer no clear-cut benefit over mechanical methods because the length of time required for the operation was not lessened and the removal of the distal cement plug in the femur did not seem any easier. As we gained experience, however, and worked with different techniques, we have refined the procedure, so that now we find it preferable to use the laser. The patients in our series were not preselected as being particularly suitable for laser surgery, so the laser was used in a variety of difficult patient problems under a variety of circumstances.

Free-Beam CO$_2$ Laser

We initially used a Sharplan 1100 free-beam CO$_2$ laser in removing PMMA. The first part of the operation consisted of the routine surgical approach. After the components of the prosthesis had been surgically exposed, moistened wound towels were clipped or sutured to the skin edges. Any shiny surfaces were covered with moistened sponges, and nonreflective surgical instruments were used throughout. The surgical team was required to wear clear plastic goggles, and the patient's eyes were covered with moist sponges. These precautions are necessary to prevent skin and eye damage by the laser. The laser armature is draped by using a sterile plastic sleeve, and the handpiece can be gas sterilized and attached to the armature during the operation (Fig. 7–10).

In total hip revisions, we usually found it convenient to remove the femoral component first. We began this phase of the procedure with a 15-watt power setting with a laser spot size of 0.4 mm, providing for a power density of approximately 8 kilowatts/cm^2. We directed the aiming helium–neon beam at the cement to be removed and activated the laser by stepping on the pedal. We used a continuous mode at 5-second to 10-second bursts. As a precaution against igniting the laser plume, we frequently irrigated the operative area with a hand-held saline spray. The products of vaporization are removed by keeping the nozzle of a high-power vacuum system

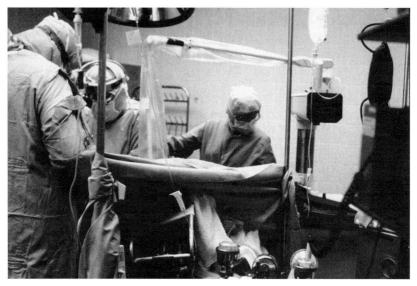

Figure 7 - 10. Photograph of the operating room set up showing the draped articulated armature through which the laser is brought into the operative field.

adjacent to the area at which the laser is directed. We have found it quite easy to vaporize all of the cement around the upper 2 cm of the femoral component by slowly but continuously moving the laser beam at these settings across the PMMA. The method is very precise and provides for no mechanical injury to the bone. Occasionally, we found it necessary to use a curette to remove membranous tissue in this area. Thermal injury to the bone can be avoided by directing the laser only on the PMMA. We also found that PMMA emits a glowing reddish color during the lasing, whereas bone emits a bright white light. As soon as the white color is seen, the surgeon should move the aiming beam. Once the cement has been removed from the upper part of the femoral component, it is usually easy to tap out the device from below (Col. Figs. 7 - 11 through 7 - 17).

Having removed the femoral component, we began the removal of the acetabular component. The laser used in the same way vaporizes the rim of PMMA around the cup. By angling the handpiece, the laser beam can usually be directed into the space between the cup and the bone to a depth of 1 cm. Frequently, it is possible to insert a curved osteotome between the cup and bony acetabulum to gently lever out the prosthetic cup. Occasionally, we used a Kocher clamp

(text continued on page 94)

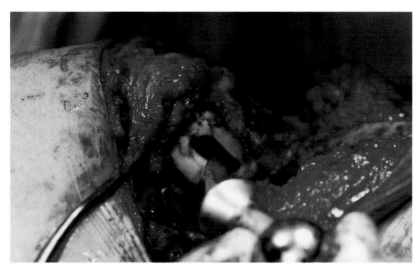

Figure 7–11. Intraoperative photograph of a loosened femoral component being removed from a femoral canal during a total-hip-revision arthroplasty. The component is completely loose in the PMMA and is easily lifted out.

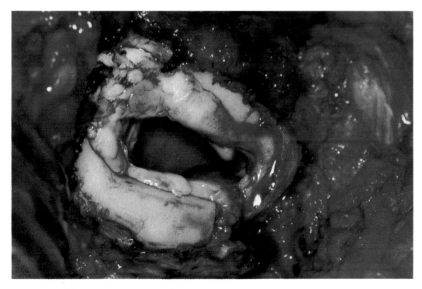

Figure 7–12. Axial view of the femoral canal after removal of the femoral component. The greater trochanter is on the left. The PMMA completely fills the canal.

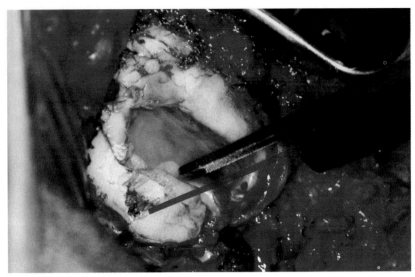

Figure 7–13. Intraoperative photograph of the CO_2 laser vaporizing PMMA in the femoral canal. The straight handpiece is on the left. The helium–neon aiming beam shows the direction of the laser beam.

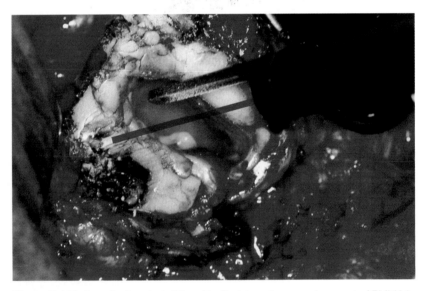

Figure 7–14. In a short period of time (1–2 min), an increased amount of PMMA is removed.

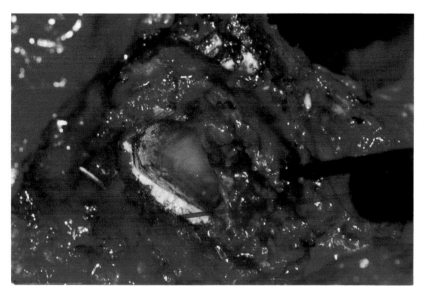

Figure 7–15. The PMMA has been debrided from the entire upper femur. Distal PMMA becomes increasingly difficult to visualize as the straight handpiece fills the femoral canal.

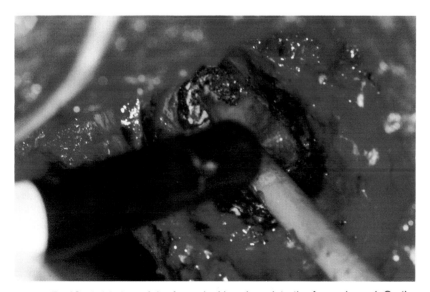

Figure 7–16. Axial view of the femur looking down into the femoral canal. On the left is the handpiece with an angled mirror directing the laser beam distally. A suction tip is seen coming in from the lower right. The laser spot manifests itself as an orange, glowing area where the laser is vaporizing PMMA.

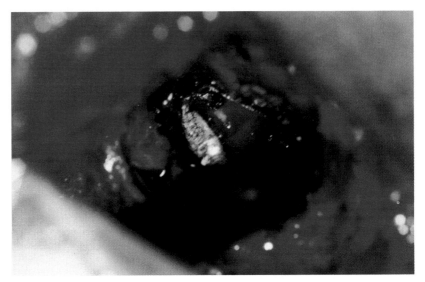

Figure 7-17. Axial view of the femoral canal. The distal cement plug is in the center of the canal, and the defocused CO_2 laser beam continues to vaporize and remove it. The angled handpiece makes it possible for the surgeon to visualize the cement plug in the femoral canal.

to provide traction to the cup during this maneuver. When these measures have appeared to require excessive force, we have occasionally cut the cup in half with the laser and removed it piecemeal. The PMMA remaining in the acetabulum after cup removal is then quite easily vaporized with the CO_2 laser.

Following removal of the two components, the laser can be used to remove or assist in removing PMMA in the distal femur. We found that the straight 125-mm or 200-mm handpieces were useful in removing proximal cement from the upper 10 cm of the femur (Fig. 7-18). Below that level, however, the handpiece blocked visualization of the distal cement, and it was necessary to approach the distal plug indirectly. This could be accomplished in one of three ways: by placing an angled mirror on the handpiece and directing the beam into the canal under direct vision while using a headlamp; by placing a laparoscope into the femoral canal and directing the laser into the shaft through the instrument; and by mounting a microscope over the femoral canal and using a joystick to direct the laser beam down the femoral shaft (Fig. 7-19).

It is necessary to maintain a constant power density of about 8

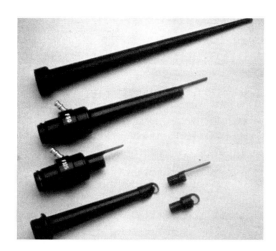

Figure 7–18. Photographs of straight and angled handpieces available for removing PMMA. On the left are angled mirrors capable of directing the laser 60 to 90 degrees away from the straight line of the laser handpiece. The handpieces have variable lengths from 120 mm to 200 mm. Straight handpieces tend to block visualization deep in the canal.

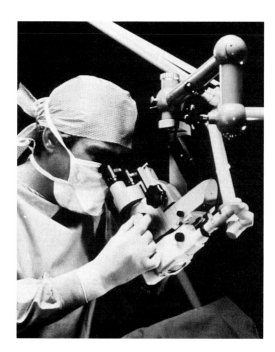

Figure 7–19. Photograph of the laser mounted on a microscope. The focal length of the laser can be controlled by raising or lowering the microscope, and the direction of the beam can be controlled with a joystick mounted on the microscope. This set-up is convenient for directing the laser beam down the femoral canal.

kilowatts/cm^2 as one works down the femoral canal. Low power densities were not as effective in vaporizing the bone cement, and high-power densities tended to ignite the laser plume. Maintenance of the optimum power density was relatively easy with the laparoscope because the laser attachment focuses the laser beam at the distal end of the instrument, where the beam strikes the working surface. In using the microscope and angled lens, however, we found it necessary to adjust the focus or power frequently. With the microscope, one should be able to adjust the focus of the beam continually as one works down the shaft and by this means maintain a constant power density where the beam strikes the PMMA. With the angled mirror, however, the focal point is fixed, and to keep the power density constant, one must increase the power of the incident beam as one works further and further down the femoral shaft. Because the power density is inversely proportional to the square of the radius of the laser spot, it is important to turn up the power setting rather quickly as one works down the cement plug in the shaft. In addition, the laser rapidly loses its effectiveness as it is obstructed by blood or smoke in the femoral canal. Effective suction and a ready supply of suction tips must be available during this phase of the procedure. The laparoscope proved useful in this regard when specially adapted with two suction tubes welded to the outside of the instrument. The laser was attached to the coupler on the top of the laparoscope, and the beam was directed through the instrument to the surface of the PMMA in the femoral canal. The direction of the beam was controlled by means of a joystick in the laser coupler. The air inflow and outflow, which is provided by this type of instrument, appeared to maintain a suitable environment deep in the femoral canal to permit the laser to function effectively in cement vaporization. We have also found that lasers can be an effective supplement to mechanical devices in removing a distal plug. If a major cement fragment disengages from the femur, for example, it is quicker and easier to remove it with a pituitary rongeur than to continue lasing. Occasionally, curettes and brushes are necessary to remove thick adherent cement membrane.

When operating on joints other than the hip, we have not found it necessary to use a microscope or laparoscope. The straight handpiece or the handpiece with an angled mirror has been sufficient because the PMMA, in these cases, is so much more accessible. The power setting and surgical technique are otherwise identical to those used in total hip revisions.

The Waveguide

We have recently begun to use a CO_2 laser fiber (Heraus Laser Sonics). The device consists of a metal-clad ceramic rod coaxial with a cooling jet of CO_2 gas (Fig. 7-20). The fibers are available in a variety of thicknesses and lengths. Angled mirrors can be placed on the tips of the fibers to direct the beam at 60 or 90 degrees away from the long axis of the fiber. The laser beam is maximally focused just beyond the tip of the fiber, and the fiber can touch the working surface without being injured. A disadvantage is that the rods are relatively inflexible, and, if they are bent, the ceramic core can break rather easily. If the ceramic core breaks, the power of the laser falls very sharply, making the device ineffective. Despite the minor disadvantages, the laser waveguides are extremely useful and appear to facilitate cement removal markedly. The coaxial CO_2 cooling jet has the added advantage of eliminating any flame-out resulting from ignition of the laser plume, because the CO_2 gas does not support combustion. The jet of CO_2 also blows blood and debris away from the working surface, making it possible for the laser beam to function with maximal impact on the PMMA and without losing energy as heat into the surrounding tissues or cement. The waveguide can be passed through a laparoscope or operating arthroscope to reach the distal plug. A camera mounted on the eyepiece of the laparoscope or arthroscope makes it possible to visualize the effect of the CO_2 laser directly as it vaporizes PMMA deep within the medullary canal of the femur. If efficient suction devices are utilized, visualization remains quite good within the femoral shaft and permits the surgeon to direct the laser down the femoral shaft with

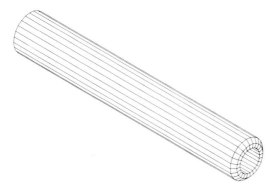

Figure 7-20.
Diagrammatic representation of the wave guide. The laser beam is directed down a ceramic rod in a metal casing. The beam is focused just beyond the tip of the rod. The wave guide makes it possible to place a precise amount of laser energy in the exact location desired.

considerable accuracy. Although our experience with the waveguide is limited, it has proved extremely useful in this application.

Clinical Data

We have performed 32 hip revisions, 4 knee revisions, and 2 elbow revisions with a CO_2 laser as our primary instrument in cement revision. Most of these procedures were performed with a free-beam CO_2 laser, and only five patients had surgery performed using the waveguide. We have reviewed the hip revisions performed with the laser for operative time, blood loss, intraoperative and postoperative complications, and length of hospital stay, and we compared these data to the same information obtained from the charts of patients who had revision arthroplasties with nonlaser techniques at our institution.

We found the laser to be extremely effective in removing cement without injuring available bone stock in the upper end of the femur. It was also useful in removing plastic acetabular prostheses and debriding the acetabulum of PMMA. Distal cement removal is more difficult, but with practice, we became able to achieve complete removal of the distal plug using the techniques noted. The recent development of the waveguide appears to be making this task easier.

There was no statistical difference in operative time, blood loss, or hospital stay between patients in whom the laser was used to remove cement and patients in whom mechanical means were used. In the group operated upon without lasers, there were two patients in whom fenestration of the bone occurred. One of these resulted in a fracture of the femur. One fatality occurred in the nonlaser group owing to a ruptured cerebral aneurysm that was not believed to be related to the surgery. During attempts to use conventional reamers and burrs as adjuncts to the laser, fenestration occurred in two femurs. We did not attribute these complications to the laser, however. One late infection occurred in the group in which lasers were used for hip revision. This occurred 2 months after a 7-hour revision in a patient who had three previous hip operations and in whom a massive proximal allograft had been used (Fig. 7–21). The infection did not appear related to the laser. As experience with laser use increased, the time required to complete the procedure was comparable to that of conventional revisions, approximately 3.5 hours to 6 hours.

The laser was also useful in removing PMMA from other joints of other patients undergoing revision. The laser beam could be directed

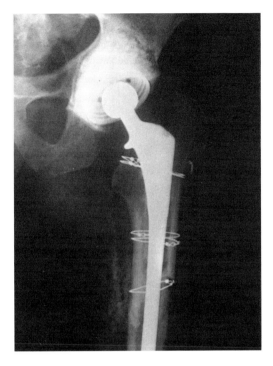

Figure 7–21.
Anteroposterior roentgenogram after removal of PMMA
by laser and reconstruction
of the hip joint and upper
femur. The laser has not ad-
versely affected revision to
uncemented prosthesis that
used allografts for reconstruction as shown here. In
38 cases, there was one
wound infection.

very precisely with excellent visualization of the working area into
narrow spaces filled with cement between the prosthesis and cortex.
We experienced no complications in four patients undergoing total
knee revisions. In one patient undergoing an elbow revision, however, there was a fenestration of the humerus in an area of paper-
thin cortical bone (Fig. 7–22).

DISCUSSION

We undertook this study because of the difficulties we had encountered in removing bone cement by mechanical methods while performing total joint revision. High-speed reamers and burrs avoided
the problems associated with the shattering impact of mallet blows,
which were necessary in the use of gouges and osteotomes, but these
devices cut through bone easily; therefore, loss of bone stock, single
or multiple perforations, and shaft fractures were not uncommon.
We hoped that a laser beam would remove bone cement in these

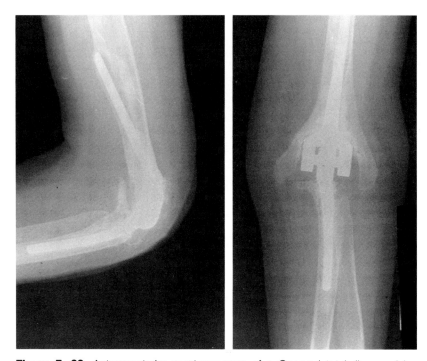

Figure 7–22. Anteroposterior roentgenogram of a Coonrad total-elbow-revision arthroplasty. Two months after this procedure, the patient fell and sustained a fracture through the ulna just distal to the tip of the prosthesis. The laser was used to remove PMMA from the ulna. It is not known whether the laser contributed to the fracture. The laser appeared to facilitate the procedure, however, by making it possible to remove the PMMA without causing mechanical injury to the bone.

patients without the risks encountered with mechanical methods. Our preliminary work showed that PMMA vaporizes 10 to 20 times more rapidly than bone with the CO_2 laser set at relatively low power densities. In addition, the thermal damage to bone appeared minimal, and the products of PMMA vaporization were removed effectively with the vacuum system.

This clinical study appears to validate the effectiveness of the CO_2 laser in revision arthroplasty. In these 38 patients, we have found that the laser very easily removes PMMA from the acetabulum and upper femur in total hip revisions and from the knee and elbow in revisions of those joints. At first, its advantage appeared to be preservation of bone stock. Initially, in our patients, it did not appear to shorten operative time, but as we have gained experience and confidence in using this new device, our facility has increased and the CO$_2$ laser is now a preferred surgical tool. Removal of distal cement in the femoral shaft with the laser still takes as much time as with mechanical devices, but the risk of penetration of the shaft appears to be much reduced. We have found that this stage of the operation is facilitated by constantly suctioning blood and smoke from the femoral canal and by raising the power setting of the incident laser beam to effective levels as one works down the femoral canal.

The use of the laser did not compromise our ability to do reimplantation of prostheses. We used allografts and cementless replantation in nine patients undergoing total hip revisions; the rest of the patients had cemented revisions. This experience has shown that the laser is a safe and effective way of removing PMMA in these cases, and after learning to use it, we have come to prefer it to mechanical methods.

Our technique for removing PMMA well down the femoral canal has evolved considerably as we gained experience. We have found that a laparoscope placed into the femoral canal provides for better visualization than is possible with the use of a microscope or hand-

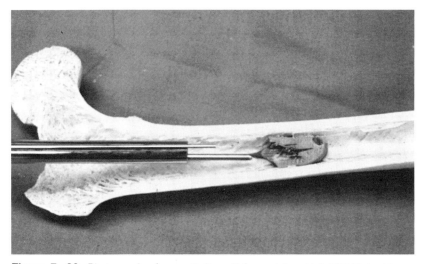

Figure 7–23. Photograph of a sagittally split femur into which PMMA had been implanted. The photograph demonstrates how the laparoscope is placed into the bone. The wave guide is inserted into the bone through the laparoscope, and the implanted PMMA is vaporized under direct vision.

piece. Adequate clearing of the working area can be achieved with suctioning through the laproscope. The laser can be passed through the laparoscope most effectively by means of a CO_2 laser fiber (Infraguide T3), so that 15 watts of power in the incident beam are delivered precisely onto the PMMA without any misdirection (Fig. 7–23). The Infraguide T3 can also be modified with deflecting mirrors to direct the laser beam in a circumferential direction. The Infraguide T3 has an advantage over the use of a free-beam CO_2 laser because the latter defocuses quickly, resulting in a rapid loss of power in the laser spot. The Infraguide T3, on the other hand, permits appropriate power density to be delivered to the tip of the laser fiber. In addition, the Infraguide T3 permits the surgeon to direct the laser beam with exact control. The joystick on a microscope or laparoscope offers better control than the hand-held angled mirror, but the CO_2 laser fiber seems superior to all other systems tested so far.

REFERENCES

1. Beacon JP, Ainsworth PM, Baird P: The carbon dioxide laser as a surgical tool for the removal of bone cement: Revision arthroplasty. Proceedings of a Symposium at Sheffield University, p 99. Oxford, Medical Education Services, 1979
2. Booth RE, Gordon SL, Carney MD: Use of the CO_2 laser in revision hip surgery. Contemp Orthop 15:17–22, 1987
3. Choy DSJ, Kaminow IP, Kaplan M et al: Experimental Nd:YAG disintegration of methyl methacrylate. Clin Orthop 215:233–234, 1987
4. Danckwardt-Lilliestrom G: Reaming of the medullary canal and its effect on diaphyseal bone: A fluorochromic, microangiographic and histologic study on the rabbit tibia and dog femur. Acta Orthop Scand 128 [Suppl], 1969
5. Feith R: Side effects of acrylic cement implanted into bone: A histological, (micro) angiographic, fluorescence-microscopic and autoradiographic study in the rabbit femur. Acta Orthop Scand 161 [Suppl], 1975
6. Horoszowski M, Ganel H, Heim M et al: Removal of cemented prostheses by CO_2 laser beam. In Htsumi K (ed): New Frontiers in Lasers, Medicine and Surgery, pp 324–328. Amsterdam, Exerpta Medica, 1983
7. Huiskes R: Some fundamental aspects of human joint replacement: Analyses of stresses and heat conduction in bone-prosthesis structures. Acta Orthop Scand 185 [Suppl], 1980
8. Krishnan EC, Nelson C, Neff JR: Thermodynamic considerations of

acrylic cement implant at the site of a giant cell tumor. Med Phys 13:233–241, 1986

9. Kroll DA, Morris MD, Norton MC: Hazards of laser degradation of methyl methacrylate. Anesthesiology 61:115–116, 1984

10. Linder L: Reaction of bone to the acute chemical trauma of bone cement. J Bone Joint Surg 59-A:82–87, 1977

11. Nelson CG, Krishnan EC, Neff JR: Consideration of physical parameters to predict thermal necrosis in acrylic cement implants at the site of giant cell tumors of bone. Med Phys 13:462–468, 1986

12. Nelson JS, Yow L, Liaw LH et al: Ablation of bone and methyl methacrylate by a prototype mid-infrared Erbium:YAG laser. Lasers Surg Med 8:494–500, 1988

13. Nuss RC, Fabian RL, Sorkor R et al: Infrared laser bone ablation. Lasers Surg Med 8:381–392, 1988

14. Reckling FW, Dillon WL: The bone–cement interface temperature during total joint replacement. J Bone Joint Surg 59-A:80–81, 1977

8

Tissue Repair with Lasers
*Overview of Tissue Repair with Lasers**

John V. White and John D. Cunningham

Tissue repair is the ultimate goal of every surgical endeavor. For more than a century, surgeons have used fine-needle and suture techniques to reconstruct tissues. Although this remains the standard method of repair today, suture material can stimulate infection, generate granulomas, and inhibit natural healing processes. However, recent unique applications of laser energy suggest that a new and less traumatic method of tissue reconstruction may be possible.

The argon, CO_2, and Nd:YAG lasers belong to the family of thermal lasers. These are instruments that emit light at a wavelength in the visible or infrared portion of the electromagnetic spectrum. Energy from these devices is converted to heat on contact with tissue, and the effects of the laser-tissue interaction are the result of this heat energy (Table 8-1). At tissue temperatures greater than 100°C, there is vaporization of intracellular water and cellular disruption. At high powers, this occurs at the epicenter of laser-energy impact and is recognized histologically as a zone of vaporization with tissue loss and cavity formation. Tissues adjacent to this area are heated less owing to dissipation of laser energy. The cells in this second zone die, but the collagen and protein matrix become fused together in an amorphous coagulum. Beyond the zone of coagulation is normal but mildly edematous tissue produced by minimal elevation in tissue temperature.

In the mid 1970s, as experience with lasers was gained, investigators began to explore whether laser energy could be sufficiently controlled at low power levels to eliminate the zone of vaporization and produce only a zone of coagulation. This was first reported by Jain and Gorisch,[1] who used a Nd:YAG laser to seal arteriotomies

*This work was supported by NHLBI Grant HL34104-02.

Table 8-1
Thermal Effects of Laser-Tissue Interaction

40°C–42°C	Dessication
43°C–50°C	Collagen expansion
50°C–60°C	Protein denaturation
60°C–90°C	Protein degradation
90°C–100°C	Collagen degradation
>100°C	Water vaporization

and venotomies in a rat model. That initial contribution generated considerable excitement in the field of laser surgery. In the subsequent decade, a flurry of research with all three thermal lasers occurred and rapidly moved the concept of tissue fusion with lasers from the laboratory to the operating room.

The wide variety of tissues fused with thermal lasers is listed in Table 8-2. Precise applications of low levels of argon, CO_2, or Nd:YAG laser energy have all been used to remodel the collagenous structure of tissue for repair. The largest experimental tissue-fusion experience has been gained with the milliwatt CO_2 laser. The superficial chromogen-independent pattern of absorption of this wavelength enables fusion of various tissues with similar laser parameters.

One of the most extensively studied areas of tissue welding has been application of this technique to the vascular anastomosis. Vascular anastomoses are subjected to constant and well-defined physi-

Table 8-2
Applications of Tissue-Fusion Techniques

Tissue Fused	Laser Used
Blood vessels	CO_2,* argon,* Nd:YAG
Gastrointestinal tract	CO_2, Nd:YAG
Biliary tree	CO_2
Ureter	CO_2
Vas deferens	CO_2*
Fallopian tube	CO_2
Nerve	CO_2*
Pleura	CO_2, Nd:YAG
Skin	CO_2, argon, Nd:YAG
Tendon	CO_2

* Clinical trials have begun.

ologic stresses. Analysis of laser fusion within this system has served not only to establish the validity of laser vascular repair but also to provide insight into the process of laser injury and healing that is applicable to other tissues.

TECHNIQUE

Pioneering efforts in tissue repair with lasers began almost simultaneously in several laboratories throughout the country. Each group developed a specific technique, all equivalent but few interchangeable. Our procedure for laser-fusion vascular anastomosis utilizes an unmodified Sharplan 1060 CO_2 laser. This instrument has a calibrated milliwatt range of 0.1 watts to 1.0 watts. Because fiberoptic delivery systems are not as yet available for CO_2 laser energy, the laser is coupled to a standard operating microscope using a microslad for precise energy delivery. The lens-focused, mirror-directed beam delivers power through a burn spot with a 420-μ diameter when mounted to a microscope with a 300-mm lens system. The invisible CO_2 beam is centered on the target area with the aid of a coaxial red helium–neon laser beam. The position of the beams is controlled with a joystick micrometer.

To create an anastomosis in an artery 1 mm to 5 mm in diameter, the ends of the divided vessel are approximated with a paired Acland clamp and irrigated with 1% Lidocaine to remove blood and minimize spasm. Three to four 10-0 nylon horizontal mattress sutures are placed to align the vessel ends in an everted fashion and create a rim of tissue for fusion. Diverting tension on adjacent sutures must completely coapt the edges.

The microscope-mounted laser is set to a power of 200 milliwatts (power density of 143 watts/cm^2) in the continuous mode. The helium–neon target spot of the laser is centered over the coapted edges, and the CO_2 laser beam is played back and forth in a sweeping fashion over the coapted edges between two retracted sutures until coagulation of the adventitia is viewed through 25 power magnification on the operating microscope. This appears as a tan discoloration of the tissue and is the endpoint of laser application. The vessel is rotated, and the second and third "sides" of the triangulated anastomosis are likewise fused. After circumferential fusion, the Acland clamp is removed and flow restored. The impact area is immediately evaluated by gross anatomical inspection and by function after clamp removal. Patency of the anastomosis is confirmed by milking a segment of the artery free of blood and allowing it to refill by blood flowing across the anastomosis. Overall, patency rates achieved with laser-fusion techniques are similar to those established for conventional suture repairs.[2] In vessels larger than 2 mm in diameter, immediate patency has been 100% and long-term patency greater than 90% with the CO_2 laser.[3]

The technique of laser-fusion vascular repair is clearly operator dependent and has a substantial learning curve associated with it. Once the skills are acquired, the time required for vascular repair is significantly less than that needed for conventional suture techniques. Ashworth,[3] experimenting on 5-mm arteries, has reported a laser repair time of 7 minutes compared with a suture repair time of 25 minutes. White[4] documented an actual laser-application time of 2 seconds to fuse arterial walls between sutures 1 mm apart. This ratio of time to distance has been constant for anastomoses in vessels up to 6 mm in diameter. Successful and efficient application of laser energy for vascular repair requires experience to recognize the visual clues that an adequate collagen bond has formed. Insufficient or excessive delivery of laser energy to the area of anastomosis can result in immediate or delayed complications.

LASER INJURY AND HEALING

The use of sutures for the creation of a vascular anastomosis remains the standard of repair. Careful evaluation of this technique reveals a pattern of both acute and chronic injury.[5] Each pass of the needle creates an immediate transmural injury that is often sealed with a small hemostatic thrombus. The fine suture frequently cuts into the flow surface as it is tightened or tied, producing a second acute injury (Fig. 8-1). The long-term presence of a nonabsorbable suture within the arterial wall may induce a foreign-body reaction or stimulate neointimal hyperplasia or other forms of disordered healing (Fig. 8-2).

Although gross inspection reveals no significant flow-surface defects, the laser also produces an immediate transmural vascular injury. This injury, however, differs from that induced by suture in that it is only acute. Light and electron microscopy have documented that the collagen bundles of the adventitia and the outer layers of the medium become reoriented and thickened, suggesting a

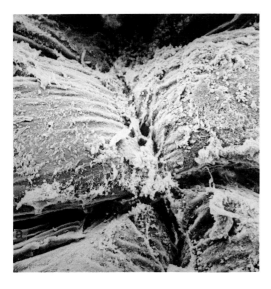

Figure 8-1. Scanning electron micrograph of a laser-fusion anastomosis 30 minutes after restoration of blood flow. The large transverse cleft through the flow surface (*a*) in the lower field was caused by a 10-0 nylon stay stitch. The area of laser fusion above this is carpeted with platelets.

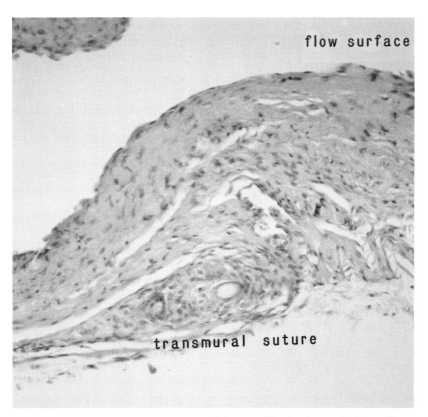

Figure 8-2. Fine sutures, such as the 10-0 nylon (22 μ in diameter) pictured here, produce a chronic inflammatory reaction.

thermal mechanism of rapid denaturation and reannealing (Fig. 8-3).[6] The protein–collagen matrix of the inner layers of the medium and the intima are completely undisturbed by the small amount of heat that penetrates through the area of laser contact. The smooth muscle and endothelial cells within these layers are much more heat sensitive and die as a result of this thermal exposure. This produces a flow surface that is devoid of endothelium but otherwise uninjured in the area of the anastomosis (Fig. 8-4). Similarly, although the medium is structurally intact, it is lacking in smooth muscle cells.

The laser produces no discernible chronic injury. The thermal effects are immediate and cause a mild to moderate inflammatory response. This response appears to target the altered collagen of the adventitia. There is little white-cell infiltration of the medium and intima. The flow surface quickly becomes blanketed with a layer of platelets without fibrin deposition. The absence of injury to the collagen structure of the intima and medium permits rapid recovery and healing.

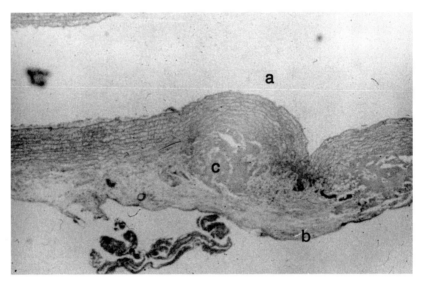

Figure 8–3. The flow-surface lumen (*a*) demonstrates minimal irregularity after laser fusion. The laser-fusion cap (*b*) gradually thickens and remodels during healing. The initial amorphous collagen coagulum (*c*) that was formed at the time that laser energy was applied persists.

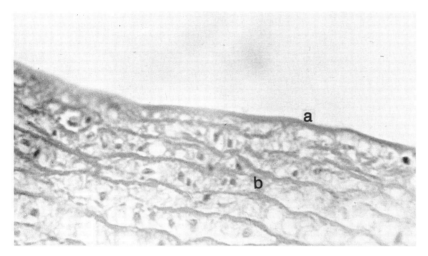

Figure 8–4. The transmural thermal effect cause loss of endothelial and smooth muscle cells in the area of laser application. The subendothelial collagen (*a*) and the protein collagen matrix of the media (*b*) are undisturbed.

Healing of the laser-fusion vascular anastomosis begins immediately after energy delivery ceases. Endothelial cells repopulate the flow surface within days of the injury. There is no significant intimal thickening. The medium remains hypocellular, with few myofibroblasts entering the area of repair (Fig. 8-5). The adventitia demonstrates a chronic remodeling process with continued deposition of new collagen in the area of laser impact. The fibrous cap forming the outer layer of the anastomosis thickens to increase the strength of the bond but remains responsive to luminal pressures. This not only reduces the likelihood of anastomotic stricture but also permits anastomotic growth during periods of host growth and vascular enlargement.[7]

The immediate strength of the laser-fusion bond is excellent, and early rupture is quite rare. Ashworth[3] failed to induce anastomotic disruption despite increasing intraluminal pressure to 300 mm Hg in 5-mm arteries immediately upon completion of the laser fusion. Tensile strength of small-artery repairs performed with the CO_2 laser was greater than hand-sewn controls when tested acutely and exceeded nonoperated controls by 6 weeks.[8] A similar study of anastomoses performed with an argon laser detected less tensile strength for up to 3 weeks postoperatively when compared with sutured repairs but no chronic difference.[2] Although the results of bursting

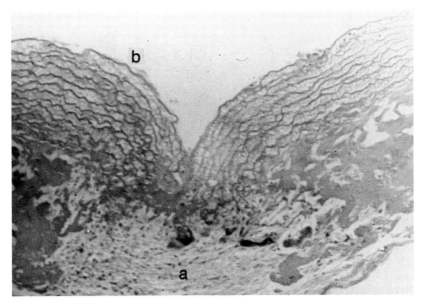

Figure 8-5. The inflammatory response is largely confined to the adventitial surface (*a*). Although the flow surface (*b*) becomes repopulated with endothelial cells, the media remain hypocellular.

and tensile-strength studies vary slightly with the type of laser-fusion technique used, each has documented an immediate hemostatic bond capable of withstanding peak systolic pressures far beyond the levels that normally occur. The bond demonstrates increasing strength over time that is consistent with the broadening of the laser-fusion cap seen on histologic studies.

Vascular repair with the laser produces a limited acute transmural injury involving the outer collagen matrix and the inner cellular population. Healing occurs rapidly without a significant inflammatory process. Cellular regeneration of the flow surface is rapid, and adventitial strength is sufficient to withstand a wide range of physiologic stresses.

THE FUTURE

Experience with vascular-tissue welding has taught us a number of valuable lessons. Foremost is the realization that immediate and long-term results of tissue repair with lasers are dependent upon both the technique and the technician. Additionally, once technique is mastered, the laser can be used with a high degree of precision to deliver energy to tissue, which results in a predictable pattern of injury and healing. Finally, the remodeled collagen induces a minimal inflammatory response and causes few adhesions.

These concepts have been applied to the repair of a wide variety of tissues. Nerve reconstruction with the laser has been reported with variable success.[9] Understandably, even slightly excessive application of energy can destroy neural function, therefore, fusion techniques must be considerably refined before consistent fusion limited to the perineurium can be performed. Sufficient experimental evidence exists to suggest that nerve repair limited to this outer neural coat is feasible and achievable in the near future.

The use of laser-fusion techniques for tendon repair has also been explored. Current techniques fail to produce a collagen bond sufficient to withstand the loads placed upon tendons. Sealing the outer layers of tendon collagen with laser energy after internal fixation, however, has resulted in healing with less scarring and few adhesions.[10]

Collagen remodeling and tissue repair with laser energy permit rapid and complete healing. As experience with laser techniques is gained, the surgeon will have within his grasp the ability to cure as well as to cut.

REFERENCES

1. Jain KK, Gorish W: Repair of small blood vessels with neodymium-YAG laser: A preliminary report. Surg 85:884–888, 1979
2. White RA, Kopchok G, Donayre C, et al: Comparison of laser welded and sutured anastomosis. Arch Surg 121:1133–1135, 1986
3. Ashworth EM, Dalsing MC, Olson JF, et al: Large artery welding with a milliwatt carbon dioxide laser. Arch Surg 122:673–677, 1987
4. White JV, Dalsing MC, Yao JST, et al: Tissue fusion effects of the carbon dioxide laser. Surg Forum 36:455–457, 1985
5. Acland RD, Trachtenberg L: The histopathology of small arteries following experimental microvascular anastomosis. Plast Reconstr Surg 59:868–875, 1977
6. Schober R, Ulrich F, Sander T, et al: Laser-induced alteration of collagen substructure allows microsurgical tissue welding. Science 232:1421–1422, 1986
7. Frazier OH, Painvin GA, Morris JR, et al: Laser-assisted microvascular anastomoses: Angiographic and anatomopathologic studies on growing microvascular anastomoses: Preliminary report. Surg 97:585–589, 1985

113

8. Hartz RS, LoCicero J, Shih SR, et al: Mechanical properties of end to end laser assisted and sutured arterial anastomosis under axial loading. Surg Forum 36:457–459, 1985
9. Almquist EE: Nerve repair by laser. Orthop Clin North Am 19:201–208, 1988
10. Herrera R: Tendon welding. In White JV, Dalsing MC (eds): Laser techniques for tissue repair. Mount Kisco Futura Publishing Co (in press)

Laser-Assisted Tendon Repair

Charles Kollmer

The goal of a surgeon treating a patient with a ruptured or lacerated tendon is to rejoin a muscle and tendon to its distal attachment in such a way that the repair is not only solid and enduring but capable of permitting the tendon to glide normally through its surrounding tissues. To achieve these goals, surgeons must adapt their techniques to the anatomical area involved. Repair of a heel-cord rupture, rotator-cuff injury, and laceration of the flexor tendon of the hand, for example, present special and unique problems and concerns.

Because tendon disruptions are common, virtually all surgeons treating injuries of the musculoskeletal system have experience with conventional methods of tendon repair and might believe that the suture techniques that they have adopted attain these goals satisfactorily. The question naturally and legitimately arises as to whether laser use would improve the results obtained. In some areas of the body, it is possible that lasers would offer little benefit. The overriding issue in many rotator-cuff repairs, for example, often appears to be finding enough tendinous tissue to reattach to the greater tuberosity of the humerus; at this time, it is difficult to see how laser use could affect this. In the treatment of injuries of the flexor tendons of the fingers or of heel-cord ruptures, the laser may, however, be of some help. In the former, the development of adhesions between the tendon and its bed most often limits the effectiveness of the repair; in the latter, the frayed ends of the tendon are difficult to reattach and frequently must be supplemented by additional tissues such as the plantaris tendon or the aponeurosis of the gastrocnemius. A technique that might solve this problem would be beneficial.

To our knowledge, tissue welding of ruptured or lacerated tendons has not had any clinical use, and there is very little reported on laboratory investigation of the subject. In an effort to evaluate its effectiveness, therefore, we performed an experiment on canine heel-cord lacerations to determine its effectiveness in tendon welding.

MATERIALS AND METHODS

We anesthetized six adult dogs and exposed the left heel cord surgically after routine prepping and draping. We transected the heel cord 2 cm above its insertion using a scalpel. In two animals, we repaired the tendon with a modified Kessler suture; in two animals, we used a 300-milliwatt CO_2 laser weld; and in two animals, we combined the Kessler suture and the laser weld. The welds were performed by directing the laser beam at right angles to the repair site. The beam was defocused slightly to produce a spot size of 1 mm. The laser was activated in a continuous mode at 250 milliwatts during the time the Kessler suture was being tightened. In the repairs performed with the laser only, the duration of lasing was maintained until the tendons appeared grossly welded (Fig. 8-6). The extremities were immobilized with long leg splints. The dogs were sacrificed at 6 weeks, and the tendons were removed for gross

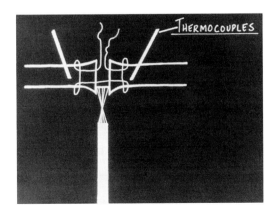

Figure 8-6. Technique used for tendon welding to augment a modified Kessler suture using a CO_2 laser. It was set at 300 milliwatts, slightly defocused, and in a continuous mode. Thermocouples in the tendon revealed temperature elevations only when the tissue began to desiccate; therefore, controlling the welding process depends on a careful visual appraisal.

and histologic evidence of healing. Hematoxylin–eosin stain was used.

RESULTS

At the end of 6 weeks, only one of the tendons had not solidly healed, that being one of the two tendons repaired with laser only. The tendons repaired with modified Kessler sutures and the laser appeared to be the best healed. They showed well-reconstituted tendon sheaths and only residual amorphous slightly stained material in the center of the tendon (Fig. 8-7, and Col. Figs. 8-8 and 8-9). The failed repair showed wide separation of the tendon ends with rounding off of the cut sutures and filling of the space between them by greyish scar tissue. The two tendons repaired with suture only showed slight separation of the tendon ends.

DISCUSSION

A milliwatt CO_2 laser appeared capable of sealing the tendon ends together and smoothing out the slight accordion effect of the tightening Kessler suture. The tendon ends appeared to melt together as this was done, provided the power of the laser was maintained at a low level. The procedure was carried out without magnification and the sealing together of the tendon ends could be visualized as it took place. The changes were subtle, however, and the aiming beam of the helium–neon laser tended to prevent appreciation of the welding process until drying of the tissues occurred so that we switched off the aiming beam once we had located the laser spot and were

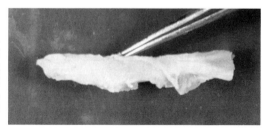

Figure 8–7. Gross appearance of the canine heel cord 6 weeks, after repair with a modified Kessler suture and a milliwatt CO_2-laser weld. The pointed forceps are at the site of the repair.

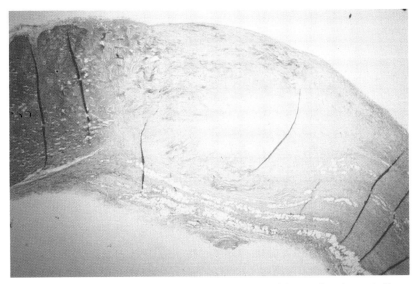

Figure 8-8. Photomicrograph of longitudinal section of the tendon shown in Figure 8-7, now stained with hematoxylin and eosin. The periphery of the tendon has apparently formed linear strands of collagen. At 6 weeks, the center of the tendon remains slightly less well organized.

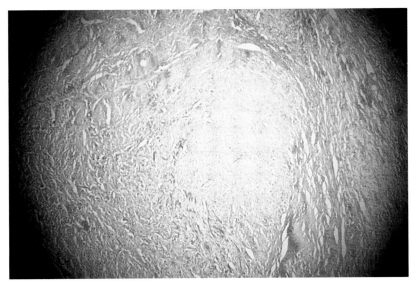

Figure 8-9. Photomicrograph of the tendon of a canine heel cord, which was shown in Figure 8-7. The Kessler suture is noted on each side of the tendon.

ready to weld. Before doing this experiment on live animals, we attempted to measure temperature changes in cadaveric tissue by placing a thermocouple 2 mm on each side of the weld. This was unsuccessful because recordable temperature changes were noted only after excessive lasing took place with drying of the tissues. Our initial study, however, seemed to indicate that tendon welding is possible. The refinement of the technique will require a different animal model, and we have begun new work in this area with flexor tendons of chickens. Clearly the weld alone is not strong enough to resist the tensile forces to which the repair is subjected, and the weld must be used in conjunction with a tension-resisting suture. The tendon weld may augment the latter, and it may also become a factor in prevention of adhesions. The need for atraumatic techniques in the repair of flexor tendons (especially in the fingers) is well known, and the laser may prove useful in this regard. The laser appears to seal the tendon wound, a property that might prevent adhesions between it and the tendon sheath.

BIBLIOGRAPHY

Partenza AB: Philosophy of flexor tendon surgery. Orthop Clin North Am 17(3):349–352, 1986

Nerve Repair with Lasers

Henry H. Sherk

Classical suture techniques in epineurial and perineurial nerves have several unavoidable disadvantages. The presence of the implanted suture leads inevitably to an inflammatory reaction that causes a cellular infiltration about the suture and the development of reactive fibrosis. The fibrotic response to the suture can be severe enough to obliterate the funicular outlines and deflect regenerating axons from a course that would lead to maximum recovery from the nerve injury. In addition, the suture defect in the perineurium or epineurium can permit herniation of regenerating fibers through the gaps in these tissues, leading to the development of a neuroma at the site of injury. Efforts to avoid these disadvantages heretofore have included the use of artificial and biologic glues or the implantation of the nerve in various types of sleeves. The goals of these techniques have been to permit the ingrowth of axonal tissue from the proximal portion of the nerve into the distal segment with maximal coaptation of a perfectly realigned nerve so as to prevent fibrous ingrowth and escape of axon sprouts. None of these techniques has been entirely successful in preventing excessive connective-tissue proliferation at the junction site or in maintaining a suitable tensile strength until healing occurs. Recent experiments on nerve repair with lasers have been conducted with the goal of avoiding the disadvantages imposed by suturing, adhesives, and tubular sleeves.[1,2]

The laser technique depends on fusion of collagen in the epineurium. Although the exact mechanism is unclear, it appears that collagen fibrils exposed to low-power lasers lose their periodicity and increase greatly in diameter. They split into fine fibrillar substructures and become closely interdigitated. The interdigitation of the collagen fibrils is the basis for the welding effect.

Several techniques have been utilized in nerve repair with lasers. Beggs and colleagues[3] described a series of experiments using a CO_2 laser with a power setting of 5 watts. The laser beam was directed through a microscope to the perineurium of the severed nerve at 0.5-second pulses and a spot size of 0.6 mm, producing multiple spot welds about the circumference of the nerve. They found that the numbers and sizes of myelinated nerve fibers in the distal segments in their experimental animals were slightly better than in those treated with nerve-suture anastomosis. They noted also that there was a greater degree of scar-tissue formation and constriction in the anastomotic zone in nerves repaired by sutures and that nerve conduction distal to the nerve injury was superior in the nerves repaired with lasers.[4]

Schober and colleagues[5] welded the perineurium of experimentally severed rat sciatic nerves with a 1.319-μ wavelength Nd:YAG laser. The laser-repaired nerves maintained their structural integrity, and there was a vigorous axonal outgrowth at the site of the lesion. Myelin regeneration took place along the axons of the distal segment.

Almquist[6] reported that repairs of epineural nerves can also be performed successfully with an argon laser. He described techniques using a minicuff of blood placed on the epineurium, and, in some cases, the perineurium, with a 0.5-second 750-milliwatt argon-

Figure 8-10. Theoretical basis for minicuff repair. The basis for the minicuff repair with argon, Nd:YAG, or KTP 532 laser lies in selective absorption of the laser energy. The blue green light will be absorbed by the blood and transformed to heat energy, and will be reflected from the white surface of the nerve, not affecting it. (Courtesy of E. E. Almquist.)

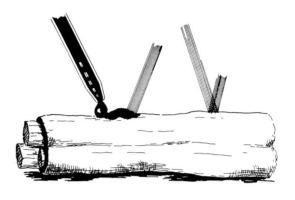

laser exposure (Figs. 8-10 and 8-11). The applied laser energy was absorbed by the drop of blood placed on the transected epineurium, and the thermal response clotted the blood to produce a homogeneous gluelike mass that adhesed the two ends of the nerve. Almquist noted "a very satisfying density of regenerated axons" in the distal segment of the nerve as well as a satisfactory return of muscle function in the rat leg 3 months after nerve repair with the laser. He noted that the potential advantage of nerve repair with lasers lies in selectively staining or tagging the perineurium about individual fascicles, then coapting and photoirradiating them to achieve an accurate internal realignment of the nerve. These techniques become increasingly feasible with high-power magnification, micromanipulators, and variable laser wavelengths (Fig. 8-12).

Figure 8-11. Repair by argon laser. A small amount of heparinized blood is placed around the fascicular repair. This is subjected to an argon laser beam, forming an adherent minicuff. (Courtesy of E. E. Almquist.)

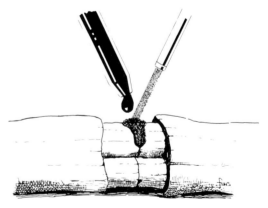

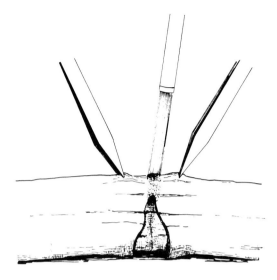

Figure 8–12. Repair by CO_2 laser. The nontissue-selective CO_2 laser beam is applied circumferentially around the nerve just enough to coagulate the external surface, resulting in a tissue bonding. (Courtesy of E. E. Almquist.)

REFERENCES

1. Boedts D: A comparative experimental study on nerve repair. Arch Otorhinolaryngol 244:1–6, 1987
2. Sunderland S: Nerves and nerve injuries, pp 533–548. New York, Churchill Livingston, 1978
3. Beggs JA, Fischer DW, Shetter AG: A comparative study of rat sciotic nerve microepineurium anastomoses made with carbon dioxide laser and suture techniques, Part 2: A morphometric analysis of myelinated nerve fibers. Neurosurgery 18:266–269, 1986
4. Fischer DW, Beggs JA, Kenshalo DL, et al: A comparative study of rat sciotic nerve microepineurium anastomoses made with carbon dioxide laser and suture techniques, Part 1: Surgical techniques, nerve action potentials, and morphological studies. Neurosurgery 17:300–308, 1985
5. Schober R, Ulrich F, Sander T, et al: Laser-induced alteration of collagen substructure allows microsurgical tissue welding. Science 232:1421–1422, 1986
6. Almquist EE: Nerve repair by laser. Orthop Clin North Am 19:201–208, 1988

Meniscal Repair with Lasers

Henry H. Sherk and Charles Kollmer

The selection of the best treatment for injuries of the semilunar cartilages of the knee has been problematical for orthopaedists in the past several years. Smillie[1] maintained that these lesions required complete excision of the entire meniscus. This point of view was, for a time, accepted by most orthopaedic surgeons, but reviews of large numbers of patients treated in this manner showed that removal of the entire meniscus almost inevitably produced late degenerative changes.[2-4] These unsatisfactory long-term results, in conjunction with biomechanical studies that clarified the important role of the menisci in load transfer,[2,5,6] led to the conclusion that partial meniscectomy was preferable to the removal of the entire meniscus. Limited partial meniscal resection performed arthroscopically has since turned a meniscal injury into a minor problem. Instead of a major open operation, the treatment of a torn meniscus needed only an uncomplicated outpatient procedure; patients were expected to return to their full activities after a short convalescence. Regrettably, however, partial meniscectomy has also been found to result in degenerative arthritis in a significant percentage of cases.[7] A poor outcome was especially likely in children and in patients with cruciate-ligament injuries.[8,9] The menisci appear to serve too important a role to be sacrificed for a short-term benefit, and a number of knee surgeons now suggest that the menisci be repaired and preserved to minimize the chances of late degenerative changes. In the past several years, many papers have appeared that present their authors' indications, techniques, and results of meniscal repair.[10-19] The issues that these papers argue are what types of meniscal injuries can be repaired and whether the repair can be done arthroscopically or through a limited arthrotomy. In general, it is agreed that the closer the tear is to the meniscal rim, the more likely the repair will succeed with healing of the meniscus. It is also generally recognized that arthroscopic meniscal repair carries some hazard,[9,20] putting the patient at risk for injury to the neurovascular structures by needles being passed out through the joint posteriorly and laterally. Some authors suggest that the procedure not be done without a posterior incision through which protective retractors can be placed,[21] and others suggest that the knee should be opened to permit the meniscus to be completely visualized as it is repaired.[22]

In this context, the possibility of a sutureless meniscal repair has obvious appeal. Tissue welding of menisci with low-wattage lasers has the potential for changing the treatment of meniscal injuries significantly and may be a reasonable alternative to either menisectomy or meniscal suturing.

Dew and associates[23] reported on meniscal repairs using an erbium:YAG laser with a 1.3-μ wavelength. The laser was used to cause coagulation and sealing of tissue at the site of experimental laceration on the meniscus with minimal tissue necrosis at the opposed tissue edges. Dew and coworkers used computer software to calculate the optimum combination of laser power, spot size, pulse mode, and time of exposure in relation to the tissue-absorption coefficient and laser wavelength. They noted the difficulty of standardizing these variables without a computer-assisted system.

We carried out experiments on dogs to evaluate the healing of meniscal tears with lasers. In our experiments, we performed knee arthrotomies on anesthetized animals to create radial full-thickness defects with a scalpel or a 1.06-μ Nd:YAG laser. The creation of the radial defect required 200 to 400 joules of laser energy. The animals were sacrificed at 2, 4, and 6 weeks, and the menisci were removed, evaluated grossly for healing of the radial lacerations, and, after fixation and sectioning, stained with hematoxylin and eosin.

We observed that the radial cuts made with the scalpel or laser healed differently. Figure 8-13 shows the lateral meniscus removed from a dog's knee 6 weeks after a radial cut was made with a scalpel. There has been no attempt at healing, and the edges of the laceration remain separated. Figure 8-14 shows the gross appearance of

(text continued on page 126)

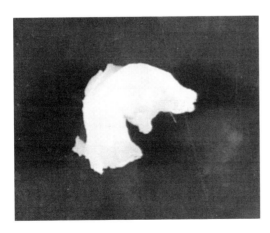

Figure 8–13. Canine lateral meniscus 6 weeks after a radial cut was made by a scalpel. There is no apparent healing of the laceration.

123

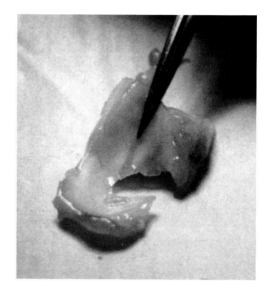

Figure 8–14. Canine lateral meniscus 6 weeks after a radial cut was made by a 1.06 Nd:YAG laser using 300 joules. The laser cut in the meniscus appears to be healing.

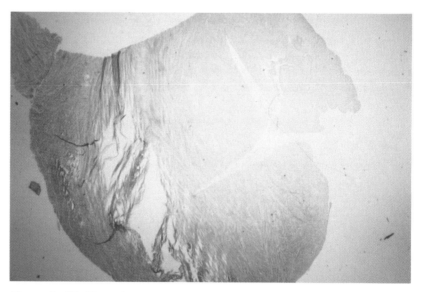

Figure 8–15. Photomicrograph of the lesion shown in Figure 8–7. The laser cut appears to be filling in with fibrocartilage, which as yet remains less well organized than the surrounding meniscal tissue.

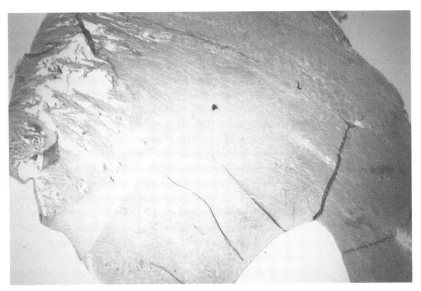

Figure 8–16. Photomicrograph of a high-powered magnification showing the boundary between normal meniscal tissue and the area of the radial defect created by the laser.

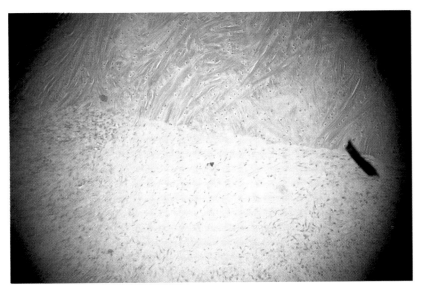

Figure 8–17. Photomicrograph of a defect by a scalpel in the canine meniscus 6 weeks postoperatively. There has been little effort at healing of the defect.

the dog's lateral meniscus 6 weeks after a radial cut was made in the meniscus by the laser. The laser cut has filled in with tissue that resembles immature fibrocartilage (Fig. 8-15). At the end of 6 weeks, therefore, it appears that a fusion and healing of the meniscus is occurring (Fig. 8-16). The difference between the healing of the cut made with a laser and that made with a scalpel is striking (Fig. 8-17).

Laser-assisted meniscal repair may evolve into an optimal treatment for torn menisci. The studies done to date show some promise in this regard, but the development of the technique has only just begun.

REFERENCES

1. Smillie IS: Injuries of the knee joint. Williams and Wilkins, Baltimore, 4th ed. Livingstone, Edinburgh, 1970
2. Fairbank TS: Knee joint changes: After meniscectomy. J Bone Joint Surg 30(3):664–670, 1948
3. Huchell JR: Is meniscectomy a benign procedure? A long term follow-up study. Can J Surg 8:254–260, 1965
4. Tapper EM, Hoover NW: Late results after meniscectomy. J Bone Joint Surg [Am] 51:517–526, 1969
5. Cascells SW: The torn or degenerated meniscus and its relationship to degeneration of the weight-bearing areas of the femur and tibia. Clin Orthop 132:196–200, 1978
6. Walker DS, Erkman MJ: The role of the menisci in force transmission across the knee. Clin Orthop 109:184–192, 1975
7. McGinty JB, Geuss LF, Mariner RA: Partial or total meniscectomy: A comparative analysis. J Bone Joint Surg [Am] 59:763–766, 1977
8. Allen PR, Devham RA, Swan AV: Late degenerative changes after meniscectomy: Factors affecting the knee after operation. J Bone Joint Surg [Br] 66:666–671, 1984
9. Lynch MA, Henning CE, Glick KR Jr: Knee joint surface changes: Long term follow-up meniscus tear treatment in stable anterior cruciate ligament reconstructions. Clin Orthop 172:148–153, 1983
10. Barber FA: Meniscus repair: Results of an arthroscopic technique. Arthroscopy 3:25–30, 1987
11. Cassidy RE, Schaffer AJ: Repair of peripheral meniscus repairs: A preliminary report. Am J Sports Med 9:209–214, 1981
12. Ghadially FN: Experimental methods of repairing injured menisci. J Bone Joint Surg [Br] 68:106–110
13. Heatley FW: The meniscus: Can it be repaired? An experimental investigation in rabbits. J Bone Joint Surg [Br] 62:397–402, 1980
14. Keene GCR, Paterson RS: Arthroscopic meniscal repair proceedings: Australian Orthopedic Association. J Bone Joint Surg [Br] 69:162, 1987

15. Rosenberg TD: Arthroscopic meniscal repair evaluated with repeat arthroscopy. Arthroscopy 2:14–20, 1986
16. Stone RG: Arthroscopic review of meniscus repair: Assessment of healing parameters. Arthroscopy 2:77–81, 1985
17. Stone RG: A technique of arthroscopic suture of torn menisci. Arthroscopy 1:226–232, 1985
18. Warren RG: Arthroscopic meniscus repair. Arthroscopy 1:170–172, 1985
19. Wirth CR: Meniscus repair. Clin Orthop 157:153–160, 1981
20. Lindenfeld TN: Arthroscopically aided menioscal repair. Orthopedics 10:1293–1296, 1987
21. Scott GA, Jolly BL, Henning CE: Combined posterior incision and arthroscopic intra-articular repair of the meniscus: An examination of factors affecting healing. J Bone Joint Surg [Am] 68:847–861, 1986
22. DeHaven KE: Meniscus repair: Open vs. arthroscopic. Arthroscopy 1:173–174, 1985
23. Dew DK, Hsu LS, Hsu TM, et al: Evaluation of lasers for use in orthopedics: Theoretical, experimental and practical observations. Scientific exhibit. 55th Annual meeting, American Academy of Orthopedic Surgeons. Atlanta, February 4–9, 1988

9

Arthroscopy with Lasers
Overview of Arthroscopy with Lasers

Henry H. Sherk and Charles Kollmer

Lasers are widely used in endoscopic surgery. Gynecologists, endo-scopic gastrointestinal surgeons, and vascular surgeons, in particular, have found lasers to be either more convenient or more effective than other techniques in their respective fields. Lasers are only beginning to be used in arthroscopy, however, and although it would seem that arthroscopic surgery would lend itself particularly well to laser usage, only a few individuals have attempted to employ lasers in this orthopaedic subspecialty. A review of the literature reveals only a small number of papers on the arthroscopic use of lasers, and the majority of these deal primarily with the basic-science aspects of lasers. Clinical reports have been rare.

Much of the original work on the use of CO_2 lasers in joints was reported by Whipple and colleagues[19], who demonstrated that me-niscal fibrocartilage healed after meniscectomy with a CO_2 laser. The meniscal tissue proceeded to a smooth, sealed margin of fibro-cartilage within ten weeks in experimental animals. In other experi-ments, these authors showed that histologically there was no alter-ation of collagen fibers or cell structure in menisci beyond 20 μ from the target site when a CO_2 laser set at 30 watts to 35 watts with shutter speeds of 0.2 seconds to 0.5 seconds was used. When the tissue was evaluated with an electron microscope,[17] there was some loss of collagen striation and organelle changes at depths of 300 μ, but these changes did not appear to indicate necrosis of the cells. Whipple and his coworkers have concluded that the 10.6 μ energy of the CO_2 laser can be well controlled with minimal side-effects. In the clinical application, Whipple and associates[16] described a tech-nique for arthroscopic CO_2-laser meniscectomy using a hand piece attached to the articulating arm of the CO_2 laser. They used the same power settings and shutter speeds employed in the experimental animals. The beam was well focused to a 1-mm spot size. It was necessary to distend the joint with CO_2 gas at pressures of 60 to 80 millimeters of mercury because the CO_2 laser beam does not pass through water. Some concern arose regarding the effect of smoke and ash on the synovial tissue.[18] There was a mild synovitis after CO_2-laser meniscectomy in experimental animals, but within 6 weeks with no joint lavage of the knees of the experimental animals, histologic evaluation showed complete resorption of carbon residue by the synovium. Whipple and colleagues[14,15] have concluded that arthroscopic laser meniscectomy may prove superior to meniscectomy done with mechanical means, although the technique remains in the developmental stage at this time.

Other authors also have described the clinical use of CO_2 lasers in surgical arthroscopy. Philandrianos[9] reported on a series of 40 patients who had arthroscopic intra-articular surgery with a CO_2 laser. In his study, Philandrianos reported 11 failures and 5 complications. He noted that the handpiece of the laser overheated in 12 cases, causing skin burns and synovial fluid leaks postoperatively. Nevertheless, he noted that the technique was developing, and he planned to continue its use. In separate reports, J.F. Smith and colleagues[12] and C.F. Smith have reported on clinical series of over 100 patients each in which they used the CO_2 laser to perform arthroscopic meniscectomies. Both have reported that they insufflated the joints with gas during laser use but that they periodically washed the joint with saline to purge the joint of carbon-ash residues. J.F. Smith and associates reported a 15% incidence of dense, bloody effusions that were attributed to synovitis due to carbon and smoke particles. The effusion resolved spontaneously. C.F. Smith, as shown later in this chapter, has not reported this complication and has indicated that his success with CO_2 lasers in the knees encourages him to begin development of CO_2 laser use in the hip and shoulder. Despite numerous problems, therefore, those investigators who have worked with the CO_2 laser in arthroscopic surgery feel that this technique has promise.

There has been relatively little published on the use of Nd:YAG lasers in arthroscopy. Glick,[5] in a preliminary experiment, found that the Nd:YAG laser (1.06-μ wavelength) was poorly absorbed by the white cartilaginous tissue and that there were thermal changes in the collagen of the menisci of a considerable (although unstated) distance from the point of laser contact. He reported that the remaining meniscal rim was unacceptably distorted and brittle. O'Brien, as shown later in this chapter, and Fronek,[4] in separate studies, have shown that the contact tip of the Nd:YAG laser effectively removes damaged meniscal tissue without producing extensive changes in adjacent tissue. Fronek's work remains largely experimental to date, but O'Brien has extended his work into the clinical setting and has operated upon a small series of patients using the Nd:YAG sapphire tip. This device, which is called the *contact laser*, converts the laser beam into intense heat at the fiber tip and functions as a heat probe to vaporize and remove tissue thermally.

Other laser effects have also been described. Srinivasan and co-workers,[13] for example, reported on the action of far ultraviolet light lasers on organic polymers such as synthetic plastics, hair, and cartilage. These far ultraviolet, or excimer, lasers produce a non-thermal effect that is different from that of the CO_2 or Nd:YAG lasers. Excimer lasers have a photochemical effect on tissue with minimal thermal damage. The tissue is destroyed by photodissociation as the laser beam breaks the chemical bond of the cell molecule. Excimer lasers therefore produce a "trench" in the tissue with extraordinarily sharp, cleanly defined boundaries. Unfortunately, excimer lasers operate in a wave length that can alter DNA. They could thus be considered to produce carcinogenic ionizing irradiation. The medium used to produce the excimer laser beam is a toxic gas, and economical delivery systems for excimer lasers are not yet available. For these reasons, excimer lasers have not been used in orthopaedics. Photochemical excimer-laser surgery, however, has the capability of removing cartilage with great ease and precision but with virtually no damage to adjacent tissue. Its disadvantages have outweighed its advantages, however, and there are no reports of its use in orthopaedic surgery.

Lasers can also affect tissue by photomechanical means in a manner that differs considerably from the photothermal and photochemical reactions noted in the preceding section. Photomechanical effects of lasers depend on the generation of extremely high energy waves for very short bursts. As a general rule, the shorter the pulse, the higher the energy. This technique is called *Q-switching*, in which laser energy is allowed to exit only in tiny pulses, between which the laser is amplified to a high peak of energy. In Q-switching, the enormous peaks of energy are released for only one billionth of a second, but the energy is so great and so briefly delivered that the tissues are shattered mechanically instead of vaporized or chemically dissociated. We were only able to find one paper describing the effects of Q-switching on cartilage. The authors (Herman and col-

131

leagues[6]) noted that Q-switch–mode Nd:YAG lasers affected proteo-glycan, collagen, and noncollagen synthesis in bovine cartilage. They further reported that Q-switching suppressed proteoglycan and collagen synthesis but that normal pulsed-mode Nd:YAG lasers stimulated the synthesis of proteoglycan and collagen. They stated that their results suggested to them that Nd:YAG-laser radiation has the potential for inducing the healing of cartilage as well as its removal.

This observation has also been made by other researchers. Abergel and colleagues[1,2] reported on the control of connective-tissue metabolism by lasers. They noted that lasers at specific wavelengths and energy densities modulate connective-tissue metabolism by skin fibroblasts both in vivo and in vitro. They found that Nd:YAG lasers at higher densities suppressed collagen production, whereas helium–neon and gallium–arsenide lasers stimulated collagen production. They noted that the modulation of collagen production may reflect the stimulation of collagen gene expression by alteration of transcriptional or translational levels of protein synthesis. Schultz,[1] Kana,[7] Mester,[8] Balin,[3] Herman,[6] and colleagues have also reported on the stimulation of wound healing and the formation of granulation tissue by varying intensities of laser energy. Visible helium–neon lasers, or cold lasers, have been in vogue for the treatment of decubiti, sprains, chondromalacia, and various other musculoskeletal conditions, but the results of treatment have not been well documented.[7,8,10]

At this time, there are four ways in which lasers are used in clinical arthroscopy:

1. Free-beam Nd:YAG laser used either with gas insufflation or liquid (water, saline, lactated Ringer's solutions) distention.
2. Free-beam CO_2 laser with a joint insufflated with helium, nitrogen, or CO_2.
3. Contact Nd:YAG laser with sapphire tips of varying shapes and sizes used in a liquid medium.
4. CO_2 laser wave guide with gas insufflation.

REFERENCES

1. Abergel RP, Yoragoya EJ, Vitto J: Differential effects of Nd:YAG laser on collagen and elostin production in chick embryo aortae in vitro. Biochem Biophys Res Commun 131:462–467, 1985

2. Abergel RP, Meeker CA, Lam TS, et al: Control of connective tissue metabolism by lasers. Recent developments and future prospects. J Am Acad Dermatol 11:1142–1150, 1984

3. Balin PL, Wheeland AG: Carbon dioxide laser perforation of exposed carnial bone to stimulate granulation tissue. Plast Reconstr Surg 75:898–902, 1985

4. Fronek J: Control Tip Nd:YAG Lasers in Orthopedics. Washington, D.C. North American Arthroscopy Association, April, 1988

5. Glick J: YAG laser meniscectomy. Presented at the triannual meeting of the International Arthroscopy Association, Rio de Janiero, August, 1981

6. Herman JH, Khosla RC: Laser (Nd:YAG)-Induced healing of cartilage. Arthritis Rheum 30:128, 1987

7. Kana JS, Hutschonreiter G, Haina D, et al: Effect of low-power density laser radiation on healing of open wounds in rats. Arch Surg 116:293–296, 1981

8. Mester E, Syende B, Spizy T, et al: Stimulations of wound healing by laser rays. Acta Chir Acad Sci Hung 13:315–324, 1984

9. Philandrianos G: Carbon dioxide laser in arthroscopic surgery of the knee. Presse Med 14:2103–2104, 1985

10. Reprinster JY, Asielaand JM, Bassleer C, et al: Treatment of primary patellar chondromalacia using a combination of quadriceps rehabilitaton and infa-red laser irradiation. Acta Belg Med Phys 8:193–194, 1985

11. Schultz RJ, Kriohnanruthip S, Thelmo W, et al: Effects of varying intensities of laser energy on articular cartilage: A preliminary study. Lasers Surg Med 5:577–588, 1985

12. Smith JB, Nance TA: Arthroscopic laser surgery. Presented at the annual meeting of the Arthroscopy Association of North America, Coronado, California, January, 1983

13. Srinivasan R: Action of far-ultraviolet light on organic polymer films. Applications to senuconduction technology. J Radiat Curing (in press)

14. Whipple TL: Lasers in orthopedic surgery. In: Shopshay SM (ed): Endoscopic Laser Surgery Handbook, pp 397–421. New York, Marcel Dekker, 1987

15. Whipple TL, Caspari RB, Meyers JF: Arthroscopic laser menisectomy in a gas medium. Arthroscopy 1, No. 1:2–7, 1985

16. Whipple TL, Caspari RB, Meyers JF: Laser subtotal menisectomy in rabbits. Lasers Surg Med 3:297–304, 1984

17. Whipple TL, Marolta JJ, May TC, et al: Electron microscopy of CO_2-laser-induced effects in human fibrocartilage. Lasers Surg Med 7:184–188, 1987

18. Whipple TL, Caspari RB, Meyers JF: Synovial response to laser induced carbon ash residue. Lasers Surg Med 3:291–295, 1984

19. Whipple TL, Caspari RB, Meyers JF: Laser energy in arthroscopic menisectomy. Orthopedics 6:1165–1169, 1983.

133

Arthroscopic Surgery with a Free-Beam Nd:YAG Laser

Henry H. Sherk and Charles Kollmer

Despite early disappointing results, Nd:YAG lasers would appear to have an advantage over CO_2 lasers in arthroscopy for two reasons. First, the Nd:YAG laser beam in the near infrared spectrum with a 1.06-μ wavelength does not "see" water. This property makes it suitable for use in a liquid medium. Because arthroscopic surgery is carried out by most practitioners with joints distended with saline (or lactated Ringer's solution), this ability to work in water is an obvious advantage. Most arthroscopists find gas distention of joints more difficult than liquid distention because of the frequent development of leaks in the joint when extra portals are used. This causes a loss of insufflation and, therefore, a loss of visualization. When the surgeon uses saline or lactated Ringer's solution to inflate the joint, the joint distention and visualization are much easier to maintain. For this reason, a laser that will function effectively in a liquid medium is preferred.

A second advantage of the Nd:YAG laser is its fiberoptic delivery system. The laser beam of the Nd:YAG laser can easily be directed into the joint through a flexible silicon fiber. This type of system provides for greater flexibility than the rigid articulating arm of the CO_2 laser in that the fiber optic cable of the Nd:YAG laser can be directed into virtually any location within the joint. Finally, the handpiece of the CO_2 laser becomes hot when there is an obstruction or malfunction. Although this occurs uncommonly, the heat can damage the skin and synovium, as has been reported by Philandiranos.

Despite these apparent advantages, we were not able to find any published reports on the use of free-beam Nd:YAG lasers in arthroscopy. Informal reports indicate that although there are some difficulties, surgeons utilizing this type of laser are encouraged. One of the problems associated with the Nd:YAG laser relates to the fact that, unlike the CO_2 laser, the energy of the Nd:YAG laser is not absorbed in the first 0.01 mm of tissue, as occurs with the CO_2 laser. The 1.6-μ emission of the Nd:YAG laser penetrates deeply into tissue, producing photocoagulation at depths of 3 mm to 4 mm from the surface. The depth of penetration varies with the amount of energy applied (joules or watts per second) and the ability of the tissue to absorb the energy. Red, pigment-bearing tissue such as endometrium or synovium absorbs the Nd:YAG laser much more readily than white, uncolored tissue such as tendon and fibrocartilage. When used at high power density in the joint, the Nd:YAG laser can effectively vaporize superficial layers of synovial tissue, but it can also produce deep thermal photocoagulation, which causes subsequent necrosis of the tissue over a few days' time. The necrotic synovial tissue would then be expected to slough into the joint; a separate procedure would be required for its removal. This difficulty has been overcome in one of two ways. Vaporization of the superficial layers of synovium with very high power densities causes deep penetration and thermal coagulation and necrosis. The tissue so affected appears to develop immediate changes in its physical properties. It becomes more friable and can be easily stripped away from underlying tissue and removed mechanically with motorized instruments. Alternatively, a Nd:YAG laser of low power density may be used to ablate only the most superficial villous synovial material. With the low power density, the laser beam penetrates minimally, coagulating and sealing the synovium. The anticipated end result would be a conversion of the synovial tissue into a flattened fibrotic scarlike layer of tissue without the sloughing of necrotic material into the joint.

Another problem associated with the use of the Nd:YAG laser in joints is the relative resistance of fibrocartilage to the lasing energy. It therefore becomes necessary to use very high power densities to vaporize these tissues, which can result in considerable heating of the water being used in the joint. Also, at high power densities, if the noncontact laser tip inadvertently touches the tissue being lasered, the tip suddenly can become intensely hot and melt the fiberoptic cable. The brass tip of the fiber can then separate from the fiber and fall into the joint. Difficulties can be encountered in recovering the small metal tips. It is possible to control these tools by performing the laser arthroscopy surgery under continuous-flow conditions, by paying careful attention to technique, and by not allowing the laser tip to touch the tissue. Sapphire tips or contact tips, which have recently been developed, may also prove useful in correcting these problems.

Our own investigation into these problems and possibilities consisted of a two-phase study. One was carried out on cadaveric human knee joints for the purpose of delineating the immediate effects of the Nd:YAG laser on fibrocartilage and synovium as well as establishing a laser arthroscopic technique. The second experiment was carried out on canine knees to determine the effects of lasers on these tissues over time and to delineate the safe and effective range of laser energy to be used in this type of surgery. The results of the animal study were described in Chapter 5 (Effects of Lasers on Tissues).

MATERIALS AND METHODS

In our experiments on the effects of Nd:YAG lasers on human joints, we carried out in both air and CO_2 gas four partial meniscectomies and synovectomies on two fresh cadaveric knees using a continuous-mode Nd:YAG laser at power densities at 30, 50, and 75 watts for periods of 2 to 10 seconds at any given location (7500 joules maximum). We completed removal of the menisci and synovial tissue with sharp dissection with a scalpel and fixed the tissues in formalin. After they were sectioned and stained, we evaluated the cartilage for the histologic affects of the Nd:YAG laser. We used hematoxylin-eosin staining for routine histologic study and alizarin blue staining techniques to evaluate the cartilage for metachromasia. We also attempted to perform the same studies on menisci submerged in saline and water.

RESULTS

In the experiment on knees of fresh human cadavers that were exposed to the laser in air or in CO_2 gas, we found that the Nd:YAG laser at all three power densities (20, 50, and 75 watts) removed the fibrocartilage of human menisci with no difficulty (Fig. 9-1). The laser could remove tissue rapidly and precisely. We could focus and direct the laser quite accurately so that the laser did not damage hyaline cartilage or synovium. The cartilaginous surfaces did not reflect the laser, at least visibly, so that the tissue apparently absorbed all the lasing energy that vaporized the fibrocartilage. The laser removed the meniscal tissue almost instantaneously over a width of 1 mm to 2 mm and at depth of 1 mm. The Nd:YAG laser, however, affected the synovial tissue differently. The laser did not vaporize synovium the way it did fibrocartilage. It puckered or shriveled synovial tissue over a wide area before the vaporizing effect became apparent. We observed this phenomenon even at high power densities. We also noted color changes in both meniscal and synovial tissue after the use of the Nd:YAG laser. The grey white meniscus turned faintly yellow where the laser contacted it, and the red synovium turned white.

When we reviewed the histologic sections of meniscal tissue and synovium that had been exposed to Nd:YAG lasers with power densities of 30, 50, and 75 watts, the microscopy mirrored the gross changes. The laser cut deep channels in the menisci and left narrow margins of tissue damage. These margins were about 35 μ wide. With hematoxylin–eosin staining, the margins contained disorganized fibrocartilage that was largely devoid of chondrocytes (Col. Fig. 9-2).

The synovial tissue treated with the Nd:YAG laser in the cadaveric knee manifested wider areas of tissue destruction than did the fibrocartilage of the menisci. The amorphous tissue debris noted where the laser entered the synovial tissue merged into more normal-appearing synovial membrane over a distance of 10 to 15 μ. In

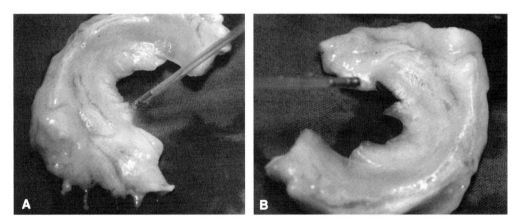

Figure 9–1. *A,* Human medial semilunar cartilage at the start of exposure to the Nd:YAG laser. *B,* This photograph shows the gross appearance of the meniscus during removal of the meniscal tissue in air with a free-beam Nd:YAG laser set at 50 watts in a continuous mode. At this high level of irradiance, the laser easily vaporizes the fibrocartilage without a discernible effect on adjacent tissue. At lower-power densities, the tissue is desiccated but not vaporized.

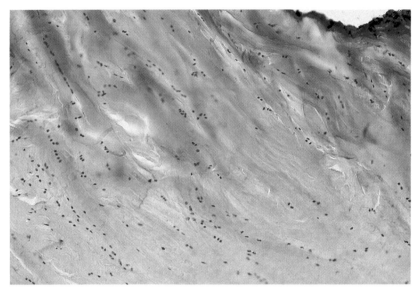

Figure 9–2. Photomicrograph of the margin of the laser defect. At the surface of the laser defect, there is a thin layer of carbonized material. The staining properties of the tissue are altered beneath this layer to a depth of 30 μ.

both meniscal tissue and synovium, a very thin line of black carbon-like tissue lined the crater that had been created by the laser. When we attempted to cut and ablate meniscal tissue submerged in a liquid medium, we found that the cooling effect of the liquid by convection thoroughly curtailed the effectiveness of the laser. It was necessary to increase the power of the incident beam to its maximum (80 watts) and double the time of exposure to obtain an effect on normal meniscal tissue at or near its attachment to the peripheral ligaments. The laser was almost as effective under water as in air in removing or cutting the edge of the meniscus and in removing villous degenerated meniscal or articular cartilage.

DISCUSSION

When we attempted to transpose our laboratory results into clinical use, we found that the free-beam Nd:YAG laser is effective under water (or saline) in smoothing villous degenerated hyaline cartilage, removing the margins of degenerated menisci, and ablating synovial tissue. It appears to change the physical property of proliferative synovial tissue so that this material can be very easily removed with a rotary meniscotome or even a blunt probe, after which the tissue can be flushed out of the joint.

The free-beam Nd:YAG laser did not seem effective in a liquid medium in removing large portions of meniscal tissue or loose bodies in a knee joint. The cooling effect of the liquid medium by convection was too complete to make this a useful modality. When we distended the joints with CO_2 gas, however, the laser became extremely effective and did ablate tissue quickly and precisely. We found it easy to evacuate the laser plume through a suction device in the arthroscope, and at the conclusion of the procedure, we flushed the joints with saline to remove any carbonaceous material. Our patients have not manifested effusions or complained of discomfort after this type of surgery.

The number of patients who have had arthroscopic surgery with a free-beam Nd:YAG laser is still small, but we feel that the technique is effective and justifies further development. It should be noted that these clinical trials are being conducted with Institutional Review Board approval only and that the Food and Drug Administration has not yet cleared free-beam Nd:YAG lasers for use in arthroscopic surgery.

The future of arthroscopy with this type of laser remains unclear. Perhaps the welding of torn menisci and the sealing and smoothing of degenerated hyaline cartilage and synovium will be done most effectively with this or a similar device. It is practical and convenient to alternate between gaseous and liquid insufflation so that various types of lasers might be used in a surgical operation on a given patient, or a single laser might be used for different purposes and in different ways. Our studies also seem to support reports that lasers have an effect on cartilage metabolism and repair, and it is exciting to consider the possibilities that a surgeon might be able, arthroscopically, to introduce a device into a joint that would have this capability.

139

Experimental Evaluation of Stimulatory Effects of Nd:YAG Lasers on Canine Articular Cartilage

Charles Kollmer

We undertook a study to evaluate the effects of low-level Nd:YAG laser exposure on chondral lesions. A previous report by Schultz[6] noted that the Nd:YAG laser had a reparative effect on articular cartilage. Our efforts were directed toward verifying this effect and also possibly defining a dose relationship in the canine model. (Our interest in this effect was stimulated by the known lack of healing noted with partial-thickness chondral defects.) Also, stimulating healing of full-thickness defects might be of value because the usual fibrocartilaginous replacement does not withstand the physiologic stress placed upon it.[2,8]

The experiment consisted of surgical exposure of right knee joints of seven dogs in which the femoral condylar cartilage was lacerated sharply, with partial-thickness defects placed on the medial side and full-thickness defects, exposing subchondral bone, on the lateral side (Fig. 9-3A and B). Varying doses of Nd:YAG-laser energy were applied to the defects (Table 9-1). The animals were divided into

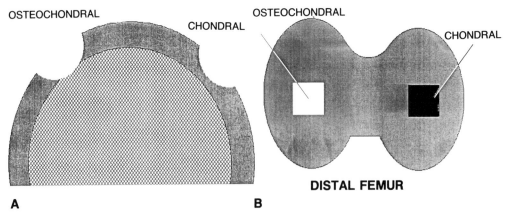

A   **B**

Figure 9–3. *A*, Diagrammatic representation of articular lesions. *B*, Representation of location and size of articular lesion.

140

Table 9–1
**Dosage Schedule of Nd:YAG-Laser Energy Used for Treatment
of Osteochondral and Chondral Defects**

Dog	Chondral	Osteochondral
1	13 joules	87 joules
2	25 joules	25 joules
3	24 joules	13 joules
4	30 joules	25 joules
5	34 joules	23 joules
6	28 joules	70 joules
7	25 joules	23 joules

three groups and placed in long-leg immobilization and 2, 4, and 6 weeks, respectively. The legs were immobilized to eliminate any healing response that might be stimulated by motion.[3,5] Additionally, the animals were pretreated with fluorochrome labeling at 1 week preoperatively (achromycin, 15 mg/kg) and intraoperatively (doxycycline, 20 mg/kg). The different tetracyclines were used because they produce different shades of yellow green under ultraviolet light.[7]

We noted minimal changes in the chondral and osteochondral lesions in the animals sacrificed at the end of 2 weeks. The subchondral bone underlying the partial-thickness defect revealed no evidence of damage from the laser exposure (Fig. 9-4), and trichrome staining of the full-thickness defects failed to reveal any ingrowth of hyaline or fibrocartilage. The partial-thickness defect revealed an apparent increase in the intercellular distance. This may represent edema, which is seen in the soft tissue surrounding laser incisions, although this is not entirely clear from these specimens.

Early healing of both the partial- and full-thickness defects was noted at 4 weeks for the 24-joules specimen (Fig. 9-5A). Some fibrocartilaginous ingrowth was seen for the full-thickness defect (Fig. 9-5B). The organization of the cartilage for the partial-thickness defect (24 joules) also showed early re-establishment of the perpendicular superficial zone. The normal palisading noted in the deep cartilaginous zone, however, is not fully appreciated. It appeared that the very low level of exposure to the Nd:YAG laser failed to stimulate any response, although those areas exposed to approximately 25 joules manifested apparent regeneration of cartilage.

(text continued on page 144)

141

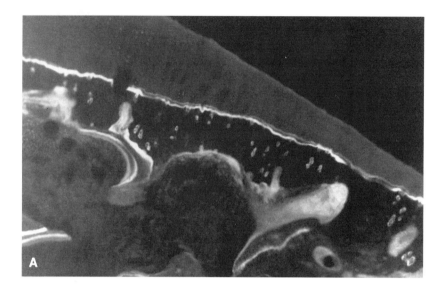

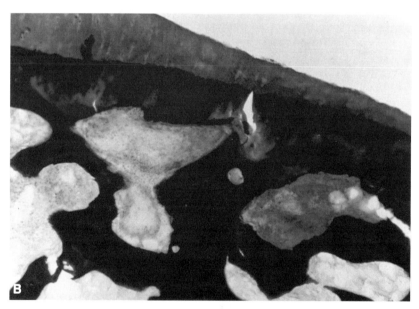

Figure 9–4. *A*, Photomicrograph of undecalcified bone at the site of a 2-week-old partial-thickness chondral defect that was treated with 25 joules of Nd:YAG laser energy and fluorochrome labeled with tetracycline and doxycycline. No damage is evident from exposure to the laser. *B*, Photomicrograph of same specimen stained with trichrome.

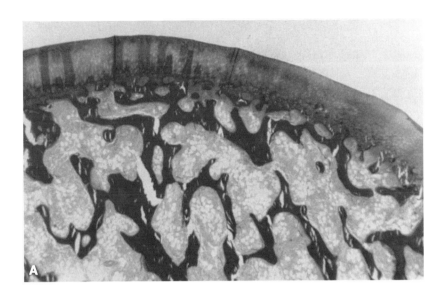

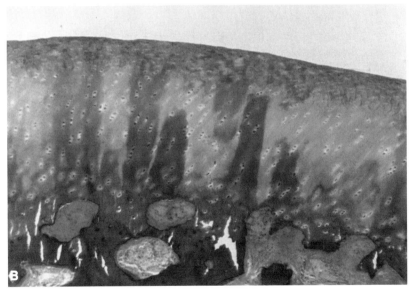

Figure 9–5. *A*, Low-power photomicrograph of undecalcified bone at the site of a partial-thickness chondral defect, 4 weeks after injury, that was treated with 25 joules of Nd:YAG laser energy. There appears to be early re-establishment of the perpendicular superficial zone. *B*, Same specimen showed at higher power showing the response of the cartilage to 24 joules.

The final group was sacrificed at 6 weeks. The joints exposed to the 25 joules also showed distinctive evidence of healing. The full-thickness defects grossly demonstrated some exuberant fibrous-appearing tissue. The partial-thickness defects had a shiny, slightly greyish appearance with some flattening of the surface. Trichrome staining of the full-thickness lesions demonstrated fibrous and vascular ingrowth (Fig. 9-6). The chondral partial-thickness defects on trichrome labeling showed reformation of the normal cartilage architecture with the tangential superficial zone, some increase in cellularity, and palisading in the deeper zones.

The nature of the cellular changes are not clear. Some preliminary investigations pertinent to this topic have been reported. Jamieson and colleagues and Reihanian and associates[4] described the dissociation of proteoglycan from laser exposure on hyaline cartilage. Reconstitution of the proteoglycan subunit is dependent on maintenance of the link protein. The link protein maintained its activity up to 70°C. Whipple and colleagues[9,10] in experiments on

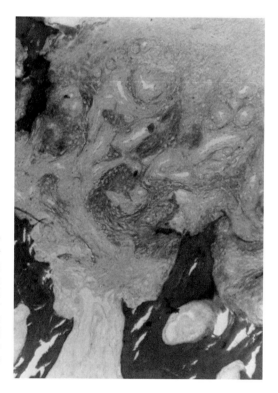

Figure 9-6. High-power photomicrograph of articular cartilage and subchondral bone 6 weeks after creation of a full-thickness defect and exposure of the defect after 23 joules from a Nd:YAG laser. There is fibrous and vascular ingrowth from the subchondral bone into the cartilage defect.

meniscal tissue, also noted multiple changes in the organelle structure of the fibrocartilage cell on electron microscopy. The basis for the laser triggering of a healing response is unclear but may have its basis in organelle or mitochondrial membrane changes and extracellular proteoglycan changes.

Although this is a preliminary study, a stimulatory effect on partial-thickness cartilage lesions could be demonstrated in the canine model. The articular response to low-level Nd:YAG lasers is apparently different for partial- and full-thickness defects. The full-thickness osteochondral defects demonstrated the expected ingrowth of fibrous tissue regardless of the degree of laser exposure. The control specimens appear as normally arranged hyaline cartilage. Harvested partial-thickness specimens revealed a definite increase in cartilage thickness and also an increase in cellular activity at the areas exposed in the 25-joule range. When higher laser levels were utilized, no response could be found. The natural history of chondral defects is that they will not heal. If the response pattern developed in this trial can be quantified, the possibility of inducing reparative responses in chondral defects with the arthroscopic use of the fiberoptic noncontact laser system appears promising. The healing response seen in acute chondral injuries might also be induced in chronic conditions, although this is only conjecture at this time.

REFERENCES

1. Jamieson AM, Blackwell J, Reihanian H, et al: Thermal and solvent stability of proteoglycan aggregates by quasielastic laser light-scattering. Carbohydr Res 160:329–341, 1987
2. Mankin HJ: The response of articular cartilage to mechanical injury. J Bone Joint Surg (Am) 64, No. 3:460–466, 1982
3. O'Driscoll SW, Salter RB: The induction of neochondrogenesis in free intra-articular periosteal autografts under the influence of continuous passive motion. An experimental investigation in the rabbit. J Bone Joint Surg [Am] 66, No. 8:1248–1257, 1984
4. Reihanian, H, Jamieson AM, Tang LH, et al: Hydrodynamic properties of proteoglycan subunit from bovine nasal cartilage. Self-association behavior and interaction. Biopolymers 18, No. 7:1727–1747, 1979
5. Salter RB, Hamilton HW, Wedge JH, et al: Clinical application of basic research on continuous passive motion for disorders and injuries of synovial joints: A preliminary report of a feasibility study. J Orthop Res 1, No. 3:325–342, 1984
6. Schultz RJ, Krishnamurthy S, Thelmo W, et al: Effects of varying

intensities of laser energy on articular cartilages: A preliminary study. Lasers Surg Med 5, No. 6:577–588, 1985

7. Simmons DJ, Kunin AS (eds): Skeletal Research. New York, Academic Press 1979
8. Treadwell BV, Mankin HJ: The synthetic processes of articular cartilage. Clin Orthop 213:50–61, 1986
9. Whipple TL, Caspari RB, Meyers JF: Arthroscopic laser meniscectomy in a gas medium. Arthroscopy 1, No. 1:2–7, 1985
10. Whipple TL, Marotta JJ, May TO, et al: Electron microscopy of CO_2-laser-induced effects in human fibrocartilage. Lasers Surg Med 7, No. 2:184–188, 1987

Arthroscopic Surgery with a Free-Beam CO₂ Laser

Chadwick F. Smith,
W. Edward Johansen,
C. Thomas Vangsness,
Leroy V. Sutter, Jr., and
G. June Marshall

In arthroscopic surgery of the knee, we use a CO_2 laser system that includes a power supply, a controller, a hand-held laser head, and an arthroscopic optical attachment. The power supply has switches on a control panel that are electrically coupled to the controller.

By adjusting these switches, we control three operating parameters: output power (P), duration of each pulse (t), and number of pulses (n). The CO_2 laser system delivers an output power of 22.0 watts for a duration (Δt) of 0.030 second and generates a dose of light energy [$\Delta E = P\Delta t$] of 0.66 joule.

Energy density is defined as the amount of energy necessary to vaporize one cubic millimeter of tissue. Energy density is determined from the amount of energy that is necessary to heat 1.0 mg of water at 37°C to steam at 100°C. The density of water is 1.0 mg/mm³. Collagenous soft tissues are approximately 80% water. Early investigators have determined that energy density for soft tissues is approximately 2.5 joules/mm.³,⁵¹,⁵² Beam diameter (d) of a laser beam measures its spot size on the surface of the soft tissue.

Figure 9-7 shows a meniscus on which the CO_2 laser system focuses a laser beam having a beam diameter of 1.5 mm. Intensity [I=P/A] of 12.22 watts/mm² is the measure of output power that the laser beam carries to the target surface area of the meniscus. Smith[47] and Whipple[50] found that arthroscopic laser surgery required similar levels of intensity (I). Figure 9-8 shows the amount of soft tissue that one dose of light energy removes from the surface of the meniscus of Figure 9-7. The incremental volume ($\Delta V = \Delta E/R$) of soft tissue is the volume of soft tissue that each dose (ΔE) of light energy vaporizes. The depth ($\Delta 1 = \Delta V/A$) of the incision into the soft tissue is proportional to the incremental volume of the soft tissue vaporized. The depth ($\Delta 1$) of the incision is proportional to the dose of laser energy, thereby making it proportional to both the output power and the duration of each pulse. For the dose of 0.66 joule of light energy, the incremental volume of the soft tissue vaporized is 0.264 mm³ and the depth of the incision for the laser beam having beam diameter of 1.5 mm is 0.15 mm. The soft tissue undergoes explosive vaporization as its water transforms to steam. Gas carries most of this steam into the cavity of the knee joint. A residual amount of steam travels into the soft tissue. We have determined that this residual amount of steam for a dose of light energy of 0.66 joule produces a zone of thermally affected, necrosed tissue of a width less than 12 μ in New Zealand rabbit menisci.[4,5]

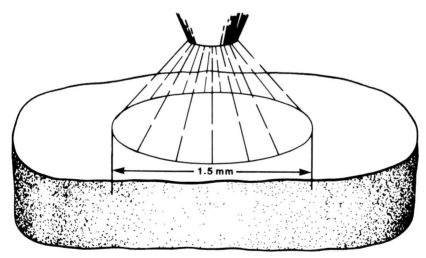

Figure 9–7. An inked drawing of a section of a meniscus on which a laser beam having a beam diameter of 1.5 mm at its surface is directed.

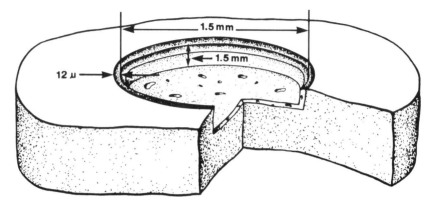

Figure 9–8. An inked drawing of the section of meniscus of Figure 9–7 showing the results of a laser beam with a diameter of 1.5 mm at the surface of the meniscus and a power of 22.0 watts for a duration of 0.030 second. The energy per pulse is 0.66 joule. The depth of penetration is 0.15 mm. (The combined total widths of carbon residue, necrosed tissue, and thermally affected, but not necrosed, tissue is 12 μ.)

Figure 9-9 is a photograph of the hematoxylin–eosin stained specimen of a meniscus processed immediately postoperatively. Figure 9-10 is an inked sketch of the photograph of Figure 9-9 that provides an improved view of the carbon residue, the necrosed tissue, and the thermally affected, but not necrosed, tissue surrounding the target tissue. The width of the carbon residue ($\delta\zeta c$) surrounding the target surface area (A) of the meniscus is 1μ. The width of necrosed tissue ($\delta\zeta n$) surrounding the target surface area of the meniscus is 4μ. The width of thermally affected, but not necrosed, tissue ($\delta\zeta t$)surrounding the target surface area of the meniscus is 7μ. The combined total width [$\delta\zeta = \delta\zeta c + \delta\zeta n + \delta\zeta t$] of the widths of the carbon residue, the necrosed tissue, and the thermally affected, but not necrosed, tissue surrounding the target surface area of the meniscus is 12μ This uniform and predictable depth of penetration appears superior to that achieved by electrosurgical devices.[8,9,20,33,39,41]

McKenzie[31] stated that the minimum width of thermally affected, necrosed tissue was 50μ. Smith[47] achieved widths of thermally affected, necrosed tissue in the range of 50μ to 100μ in 114 clinical cases.[47] He had significant effusions in 42 cases. Whipple achieved widths of thermally affected, necrosed tissue in the range of 20μ to 50μ[50,51,52,53,54] in ten cadaveric knee joints. We have found thermally affected, necrosed meniscal tissue in the range of 10μ to 12μ in 192

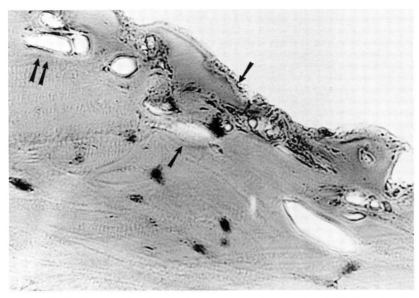

Figure 9–9. Photograph of a specimen of a meniscus stained with hematoxylin and eosin that was taken immediately postoperatively at a magnification of 4000. In this photograph, a line of 1.3 inches is drawn to represent 8 μ. The pair of upper arrows indicates the thermally affected tissue. The pair of lower arrows indicates normal tissue.

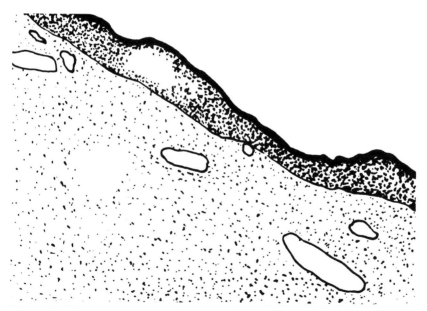

Figure 9–10. An inked drawing of the photograph of Figure 9–9 showing the zone of carbonization, the zone of tissue necrosis, and the zone of heat-affected tissue.

149

clinical cases. None of our patients had effusions that required aspiration (Table 9-2). We attribute this to the fact that the zone of thermally affected necrosed tissue is so narrow and we hypothesize that the smaller the width of thermally affected, necrosed tissue, the fewer the incidences of effusions and tissue reaction.

CHONDRAL AND SYNOVIAL KNEE SURGERY

Our study comparing results of arthroscopic laser surgery for partial meniscectomy with nonlaser controls began in January of 1985. It has involved preselection of patients with primary meniscal problems and no significant ligamentous instability. Many of these patients had undergone previous surgery (22%). Although the primary problems were meniscal, we have treated 92% of the patients by laser vaporization for grade 2 through grade 4 chondromalacic lesions at either the patella or the femur. Some of the patients (18%) underwent limited partial synovectomy. The primary goal of the study was to determine the safety and efficacy of the arthroscopic laser system and document any significant complications that might ensue. Fortunately, the complications have compared favorably with historical controls.[1,28] The combination of procedures, however, does not allow for the deduction of hard data in relation to the comparative results of standard and laser arthroscopic surgery for either chondroplasty or partial synovectomy. The technical ease of the procedure and the initial results have been encouraging, however. Four follow-up video examinations have also shown excellent chondral contour. Light and electron microscopy indicate a high-level

Table 9–2

Complications in 192 Knee Arthroscopies Performed with a Free-Beam CO_2 Laser

Complications	Percentage	No. of Cases
Death	0	0
Arthrotomy	0	0
Effusions requiring aspiration	0	0
Phlebitis requiring treatment	0.5	1
Widened incisions (0>2.5 cm)	13	25
Subcutaneous emphysema	100	192

fibrocartilaginous response that does not become true hyaline cartilage. Other authors have indicated that the laser causes replication
of cartilage cells.[24,32,35]

Arthroscopic synovectomy, although still controversial, compares
favorably in completeness with standard synovectomy and probably
offers less morbidity.[1,2,13,22,25-27,29,32,43] The theoretical advantage of
the gated CO_2 laser system in more routine arthroscopic surgery led
us to compare laser arthroscopic synovectomy with standard open
synovectomy and standard arthroscopic synovectomy.

We have already mentioned the advantages of laser chondroplasty (technical effectiveness, efficiency, possible cell replication,
and a controllable depth of incision). Because there are variable
etiologies of chondromalacia patellae, including recurrent subluxa-
tion, congenital deformity, trauma, patella alta, patella baja, and
idiopathic chondromalacia, and because there is difficulty in gauging
subjective response to therapy, the recommendations for treatment
in the literature have varied from exercises to patellectomy to surface replacement.[10,16,30,36] The low morbidity from arthroscopic-laser
chondroplasty and the positive subjective responses of the patients
have encouraged us to continue our use of the CO_2 laser for these
purposes.

Technique for Arthroscopic Laser
Surgery of the Knee

The technique for arthroscopic laser surgery of the knee is identical
to any other arthroscopic surgery at the knee, with the following
exceptions. The utilization of a gaseous environment improves the
efficiency of the CO_2 laser system, and we believe that the CO_2 laser
system is the most effective in the knee because of the high water
content of the structures within the knee. We have utilized helium,
CO_2, and nitrogen, but we prefer CO_2 because of its effectiveness as
a coolant agent and its ready absorbability. The suction device must
be utilized to evacuate the plume that results from vaporization of
the target tissue. Carbonization is a normal by-product of the vaporization process in laser surgery, and must be evacuated by mechanical and aqueous debridement following use of the laser. Depending
on the pressure of gas that is utilized (from 0.25 psi to 2.0 psi),
subcutaneous emphysema may be a transient by-product of laser
arthroscopic surgery of the knee; therefore, a tourniquet is recommended to restrict the extent of subcutaneous emphysema.

A tourniquet is utilized, and two inferior and one superior standard arthroscopic incisions are required. The diagnostic arthroscopy is undertaken in a gaseous environment with the gas afferent at the arthroscope (Col. Fig. 9-11). When arthroscopic laser surgery is undertaken, the afferent gas tube is transferred to the laser, and laser surgery is undertaken at the target tissue. Suction is utilized either through the arthroscope or, in more extensive cases, through a separate incision. On completion of the laser procedure, the water afferent at the superior entry portal is opened and lavage is undertaken at the target area with manual debridement. On completion of this procedure, a diagnostic evaluation is undertaken. If further laser surgery is necessary, suction is utilized to evacuate the aqueous environment and the gaseous environment is re-established. (In the CO_2 laser system that I utilize, there is a special "Y tube" that facilitates the rapid alternation between aqueous and gaseous environment in a few seconds.) On completion of the procedure, standard closure is undertaken. The patient may bear weight to tolerance but should be warned of the possibility of transient subcutaneous emphysema.

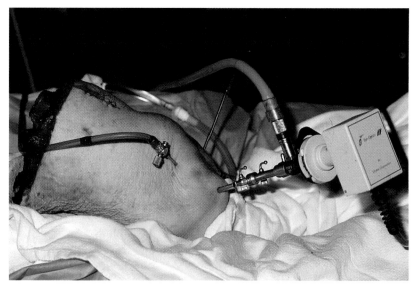

Figure 9-11. Surgical arthroscopy using a CO_2 laser. The laser has been inserted into the joint, which has been inflated with CO_2 gas. A tourniquet is always used.

ARTHROSCOPY OF THE SHOULDER JOINT

Diagnostic and therapeutic arthroscopy of the shoulder joint is now an accepted procedure. Andrews[3,4] has popularized the technique. He has reported favorable short-term results in a population with high needs and high expectations. Sixty-four per cent of the patients were baseball pitchers whose average duration of symptoms was 12 months. These patients commonly had pain with overhead activities and had negative arthrograms with full range of motion and no atrophy. The most common lesion that he found at diagnostic arthroscopy was a partial rupture of the rotator cuff. Following debridement by standard methods, 85% of the patients returned satisfactorily to their preoperative athletic activities. We have extended the concept of diagnostic and standard shoulder arthroscopic surgery to laser arthroscopic surgery. The arthroscopic laser system superficially vaporizes lesions with high surface area and low volume, which are typical of degenerative cartilaginous and collagenous lesions. With this concept in mind, we undertook laser debridement of 12 cadaveric shoulders.[44] The technique seems safe and effective, but in our first endeavor on a human shoulder, helium gas caused 24 hours of subcutaneous emphysema at the neck and scrotum. Although the complication was only transient and the 6-month results were satisfactory, we now feel that, in the shoulder joint, diagnostic arthroscopy should be performed in a saline environment and the arthroscopic laser surgery in a gas environment, preferably CO_2, for a period limited to 15 minutes. At this time, we are not continuing laser arthroscopy of the shoulder.

ARTHROSCOPY OF THE WRIST, ELBOW, AND ANKLE JOINT

The indications for arthroscopic surgery of the elbow, wrist, and ankle joints are removal of loose bodies, treatment of osteochondritis dissecans, synovectomy for nonspecific and rheumatoid synovitis, treatment of certain simple fractures, debridement of degenerative arthritis, excision of osteophytes, and, occasionally, evaluation and treatment of the undiagnosed painful joint.[5-7,11,12,14,15,21,28,37,38] The common clinical degenerative problems that standard arthroscopic techniques treat present with high surface area, low volume, and high water content. These lesions are ideal for laser therapy. We confirmed this thesis in 12 cadaveric elbows.[44] The gross and microscopic cadaveric success led to clinical evaluations. A multicenter study is now under an investigational device exemption (IDE) pending final approval from the Food and Drug Administration (FDA).

LASER FUSION

Repair of structures by tissue welding with a laser has been technically feasible for 10 years; however, surgeons have only studied the procedure in depth for the past 7 years. Most of these surgeons have found the strength of the collagen weld to be insufficient.[19,46] Dew[17,18] appears to have solved the problem of aneurysm formation and disruption with an Erb:YAG laser system. More work must be done, however, before laser fusion can be considered to be a standard and routine procedure. In our work with repair of menisci with a CO_2 laser system, the strength of the bond has been inadequate[46] and has not surpassed that achieved by conventional techniques.[23,34,40]

CONCLUSIONS

We have performed arthroscopic laser surgery in 525 knee joints between January 1985 and March 1988, using a CO_2 laser in joints distended with CO_2 gas. We have noted no lasting complications. The results have been good, and we believe that the laser technique for knee arthroscopy is safe and effective.

Recently, there has been an increased interest in performing arthroscopic surgical procedures on other joints.[5,6,7,11,12,14,15,21,28,37,38] We have performed arthroscopic laser surgery on multiple "non-knee" joints of cadavers and have now initiated a multicenter trial for arthroscopic laser surgery on the elbow, wrist, shoulder, and ankle joints. We feel that the CO_2 laser is an effective, efficient, and safe tool for use in arthroscopy.

REFERENCES

1. Altman RD, Kates J: Arthroscopy of the knee. Semin Arthritis Rheum 13, No. 7:188–199, 1983

2. Altman RD, Gray R: Diagnostic and therapeutic uses of the arthroscope in rheumatoid arthritis and osteoarthritis. Am J Med 75:50–55, 1983

3. Andrews JR, Carson WG: Shoulder joint arthroscopy. Orthopedics 6, No. 9:1157–1162, 1983

4. Andrews JR, Broussard TS, Carson WG: Arthroscopy of the shoulder in the management of partial tears of the rotator cuff: A preliminary report. Arthroscopy 1, No. 2:117–122, 1985

5. Andrews JR, Carson WG: Arthroscopy of the elbow. Arthroscopy 1, No. 2:97–107, 1985

6. Andrews JR, Previte WJ, Carson WG: Arthroscopy of the ankle: Technique and normal anatomy. Foot Ankle 6, No. 1:29–33, 1985

7. Andrews JR, St. Pierre RK, Carson WG: Arthroscopy of the elbow. Clin Sports Med 5, No. 4:653–662, 1986

8. Aritomi H: Arthroscopic synovectomy of the knee joint with the electric resectoscope. Scand J Haematol (Suppl 40) 33:249–262, 1984

9. Balduini FC, Peff TC, Torg JS: Application of electrothermal energy in arthroscopy. Arthroscopy 1, No. 4:259–263, 1985

10. Bentley G, Dowd G: Current concepts of etiology and treatment of chondromalacia patellae. Clin Orthop Rel Res, No. 189:209–228, 1984

11. Boe S: Arthroscopy of the ankle joint. Arch Ortho Trauma Surg, 105:285, 1986

12. Bora FW, Osterman AL, Maitin E, et al: The role of arthroscopy in the treatment of disorders of the wrist. Contemp Orthop 12, No. 4:28–36, 1986

13. Casscells CD: Commentary: The argument for early arthroscopic synovectomy in patients with severe hemophilia. J Arthros Rel Surg 3(2):78–79, 1987

14. Chen Y-C: Arthroscopy of the wrist and finger joints. Orthop Clin North Am 10, No. 3:723–733, 1979

15. Cofield RH: Arthroscopy of the shoulder. Mayo Clin Proc 58:501–508, 1983

16. Dandy DJ: Abrasion chondroplasty. Arthroscopy 2, No. 1:51–53, 1986

17. Dew DK: Laser-assisted microsurgical research (with panel discussion on microsurgery and laser). Faculty/University of Miami postgraduate course on New Technology in Orthopaedics and Rehabilitation, Bal Harbor, Florida, December, 1982

18. Dew DK, Lo HK: Carbon dioxide laser microsurgical repair of soft tissue: Preliminary Observations. Presented at the American Society for Laser Medicine and Surgery, New Orleans, Louisiana, January, 1983

19. Dew DK, Verdeia JC: Carbon dioxide laser repair of rat sciatic nerves. Presented at the Eastern Student Research Forum, Miami, Florida, March, 1983

20. Fox JM, Ferke RD, DelPizzo W, et al: Electrosurgery in orthopaedics: Part II — Applications to arthroscopy. Contemp Orthop 8, No. 2:37–44, 1984

21. Guhl JF: Arthroscopy and arthroscopic surgery of the elbow. Orthopedics 8, No. 10:1290–1926, 1985

22. Hefti F, Morscher E, Koller F: The use of laser beams for operations in haemophilia. Scand J Haematol (Suppl 40) 33:281–289, 1984

23. Henning CE, Lynch MA, Clark JR: Vascularity for healing of meniscus repairs. Arthroscopy 3, No. 1:13–18, 1987

24. Herman JH, Khosla RC: Laser (Nd:YAG)-induced healing of cartilage. Arthritis Rheum 30, No. 4:S128, 1987

25. Highgenboten CL: Arthroscopic synovectomy. Arthroscopy, 1, No. 3:190–193, 1985

26. Highgenboten CL: Arthroscopic synovectomy. Orthop Clin North Am 13, No. 2:399–405, 1982

27. Horoszowski H, Heim M, Seligsohn U, et al: Use of the laser scalpel in orthopaedic surgery on the haemophilic patient, pp 189–193. In Haemophilia. Tumbridge House, England, Castle House Publications, Chapter 24, 1981

28. Jackson RW: Current concepts review — arthroscopic surgery. J Bone Joint Surg 65-A, No. 3:416–420, 1983

29. Limbard TJ, Dennis SC: Synovectomy and continuous passive motion (CPM) in hemophiliac patients. J Arthrosc Rel Surg 3, No. 2:74–77, 1987

30. McCarroll JR, O'Donoghue DA, Grana WA: The surgical treatment of chondromalacia of the patellae. Clin Orthop Rel Res, No. 175:130–134, 1983

31. McKenzie AL: How far does thermal damage extend beneath the surface of CO_2 laser incisions? Phys Med Biol 28:905–912, 1983

32. Meyers JF: Surgical technique for arthroscopic synovectomy. Contemp Orthop 10, No. 5:41–45, 1985

33. Miller GK, Drennan DB, Maylahn DJ: The effect of technique on histology of arthroscopic partial meniscectomy with electrosurgery. Arthroscopy 3, No. 1:35–44, 1987

34. Morgan CD, Casscells BW: Arthroscopic meniscus repair: A safe approach to the posterior horns. Arthroscopy 2, No. 1:3–12, 1986

35. Norton LA: Effects of a pulsed electromagnetic field on a mixed chondroblastic tissue culture: Section III — basic science and pathology. Clin Orthop Rel Res No. 167:280–290, 1982

36. Ogilvie-Harris DJ, Jackson RW: The arthroscopic treatment of chondromalacia patellae. J Bone Joint Surg 66-B, No. 5:660–665, 1984

37. Parisien JS, Vangsness T: Operative arthroscopy of the ankle: Three years' experience. Clin Orthop Rel Res 199:45–63, 1985

38. Parisien SJ: Arthroscopic treatment of osteochondral lesions of the talus. Am J Sports Med 14, No. 3:211–217, 1986

39. Rand JA, Gaffey TA: Effect of electrocautery of fresh human articular cartilage. Arthroscopy 1, No. 4:242–246, 1985
40. Rosenberg TD, et al: Arthroscopic meniscal repair evaluated with repeat arthroscopy. Arthroscopy 2, No. 1:14–20, 1986
41. Schosheim PM, Caspari RB: Evaluation of electrosurgical meniscectomy in rabbits. Arthroscopy 2, No. 2:71–76, 1986
42. Schultz RJ, Krishnamurthy S, Theimo W, et al: Effects of varying intensities of laser energy on articular cartilage. Lasers Surg Med 5, No. 4:577–588, 1985
43. Shibata T, Shiraoka K, Takubo N: Comparison between arthroscopic and open synovectomy for the knee in rheumatoid arthritis. Arch Ortho Trauma Surg, No. 105:257–262, 1986
44. Smith CF, Johansen WE, Vangsness CT, et al: Does success of arthroscopic laser surgery in the knee joint warrant its extension to "non-knee" joints? SPIE Lasers Med 712:214–217, 1986
45. Smith CF, Marshall GJ, Snyder SJ, et al: Comparisons of tissue effects of a surgical scalpel, an electrocautery apparatus and a carbon dioxide laser system when used for making incisions into the menisci of New Zealand rabbits. Lasers Surg Med 3:305–369, 1984
46. Smith CF, Johansen WE, Sutter LV, et al: Meniscal repair utilizing a hand-held carbon dioxide laser. Poster exhibited at the annual meeting of the American Academy of Orthopaedic Surgeons, San Francisco, California, January, 1987
47. Smith JB, Nance T: Laser energy in arthroscopic surgery (unpublished data)
48. Verschueren RCJ: Thermal damage in adjoining tissues after using the focused CO_2 laser beam. In The CO_2 Laser in Tumor Surgery. Amsterdam, Van Gorcum, 1976
49. Verschueren RCJ: Tissue reaction to the CO_2 laser in general. In Microscopic and Endoscopic Surgery with the CO_2 Laser. Boston, John Wright, 1982
50. Whipple TL, Caspari RB, Meyers JF: Arthroscopic meniscectomy by CO_2 laser vaporization in a gas medium. Orthop Trans 6, No. 1:136, 1982
51. Whipple TL, Caspari RB, Meyers, JF: Arthroscopic laser meniscectomy in a gas medium. Arthroscopy 1, No. 1:2–7, 1985
52. Whipple TL, Caspari RB, Meyers JF: Laser energy in arthroscopic meniscectomy. Orthopaedics 6, No. 9:1165–1169, 1983
53. Whipple TL, Caspari RB, Meyers JF: Laser subtotal meniscectomy in rabbits. Lasers Surg Med 3:297–304, 1984
54. Whipple TL, Caspari RB, Meyers JF: Synovial response to laser-induced carbon ash residue. Lasers Surg Med 3:291–295, 1984

Arthroscopic Surgery with a Contact Nd:YAG Laser

Anne M. Kelly,
Stephen J. O'Brien,
Drew V. Miller,
Stephen V. Fealy, and
Russell F. Warren

The advent of arthroscopy was accompanied by a need for instrument development and technical adaptations. As with any concept as revolutionary as arthroscopy, there were many skeptics. In fact, the initial interest in what was called *arthroendoscopy* in 1921 had waned by the mid 1930s owing to lack of technologic resources. Not until the 1950s, when Dr. Masaki Watanabe created the first practical arthroscope, did it become obvious that arthroscopy was not a passing fad.

Since the 1970s, arthroscopists have been challenged by the need for adaptation of existing cutting and dissecting tools for effective use in arthroscopy. Instruments were needed that were capable of working inside a specific joint space. In addition, instruments had to be developed that could be introduced into the joint through arthroscopy portals. Generally, these instruments were 3 mm to 4 mm in diameter. Instruments also had to maintain a degree of maneuverability upon being introduced into the joint.

Of course, arthroscopy is no longer in its infancy, and many of the problems just mentioned have been minimized by advanced instrumentation; however, many of the instruments that have been developed to date share several common problems. In addition to the difficulty encountered in introducing the instrument through an arthroscopy portal, there are problems with opening and closing of the instrument in a tight compartment, which can cause damage to the surrounding articular surfaces.

Several studies have made broad evaluations regarding the use of the noncontact CO_2 laser in arthroscopic procedures. The CO_2 laser utilizes lenses to adequately converge its rays to a point. Problems with the delivery of the energy from a CO_2 laser are a consequence of the wavelength of CO_2 laser radiation. Its wavelength is not only absorbed by water but by glass as well. As a result, the energy beam cannot be transmitted over great distances through contemporary fibers, rather, the beam must be reflected through a system of mirrors and conduits to bend it.[1]

Another problem with using CO_2 laser in arthroscopy is that the saline medium used to inflate the joint (as well as to cool thermal effects) cannot remain in the joint when a CO_2 laser is operating. Whipple[2] conducted trials with air, oxygen, CO_2, nitrous oxide, and nitrogen as means of joint distention. In his experiment, which involved meniscectomy with CO_2 laser vaporization, nitrogen was chosen as the insufflation medium because of its physiologic and physiochemical properties as well as its compatibility with the transmission of CO_2-laser wavelengths. Concern exists about proper heat dissipation without a fluid medium.[3]

Finally, with the CO_2 laser, all target surfaces within the joint must be dried in order for the tissue itself to absorb the energy. Whipple also found that heat was conducted radially from the surface through the water contained in the fibrocartilage.

The following are two distinct disadvantages of the CO_2 laser in arthroscopy: first, there are no lenses capable of transmitting CO_2-laser wavelengths (10.6μ of radiation), which necessitates the introduction of an additional attachment (articulated arm) via a separate portal; and second, the inability to transmit 10.6μ of radiation from a CO_2 laser through water or saline requires distention of the joint with a gas medium.[4]

Many studies have involved the application of electrothermal energy (electrocautery) to arthroscopy. Here again several problems are encountered. Owing to its high conductivity, saline medium is inappropriate in electrocautery arthroscopic procedures. Several investigators chose sterile water as a distention medium, however, problems do exist with this choice. Although Fox and coworkers[3] switch the medium only briefly during electrocautery use, it does not appear to be a physiologic medium. Rand[5] found that, in rabbits, lavage of the joint with sterile water resulted in a decrease in synovial-cell integrity and an abnormal appearance of the articular cartilage. Although the sterile water does provide a stable solution for electrothermal energy, it does not support proteoglycan synthesis, and its hypo-osmolarity leads to rapid absorption and chondrocyte swelling. Snyder[6] recommends the use of a glycerol-based solution for irrigation during arthroscopy. Based on tests he has conducted, it seems a more appropriate medium than sterile water and other nonconductive solutions.

Another problem with electrocautery is the technique that is recommended by Fox and coworkers[3] for best cutting results. They describe the delivery method as "throwing a wave" in front of the electrode tip (by activating the electrode just prior to touching the tissue) with the tip held approximately 1 mm from the tissue to be incised. Such a modification in delivery could lead to widely varying results depending upon the surgeon delivering the electrothermal energy.

Thermal burns have also been a problem with electrocautery procedures. Whether resulting from loss of contact with the grounding pad or an increase in current density in too small an area (or even an active electrode tip contacting skin) burns seem more frequent a problem with electrocautery than with other devices available.

Electrocautery settings have been reported in the 30-watt to 50-watt range in various studies.[7] In studies we recently performed at our institution, these wattage settings lead to full-thickness lesions in articular cartilage with a large lateral margin of necrosis. Balduini[7] also found that once the instrument penetrated the meniscal tissue, it produced scarification of the tibial articular surface. Histologically, the increased wattage setting results in a very well defined zone of thermal damage that can be visualized with trichrome stain.[8]

The disadvantages inherent in CO_2 laser and electrocautery arthroscopy can be overcome with the contact Nd:YAG laser. Its ability to transmit in saline medium facilitates its use in arthroscopic procedures. Additionally, because it is a *contact* laser, its energy is more precisely focused and the resulting lateral necrosis is minimized. Finally, with the appropriate delivery fibers, access to tight spaces, which are so often encountered in arthroscopy, is more easily obtained. For these reasons, we chose to evaluate the efficiency of the Nd:YAG laser in comparison to that of electrocautery. The standard scalpel was used as a control in all instances.

The contact Nd:YAG laser (Surgical Laser Technologies, Malvern, Pennsylvania) includes three attachments: gas–fluid cartridge, fiber delivery system, and tip. The cartridge is a standard attachment and is inserted into an opening on the top of the laser (Fig. 9-12). There are several types of delivery fibers (Fig. 9-13). The selection becomes important in the clinical studies to facilitate entry through an arthroscopy portal.

The first phase of our study involved the use of canine and fresh frozen cadaveric knees. The purpose of this initial step was to determine the proper wattage, fiber, and tip for further studies. Following

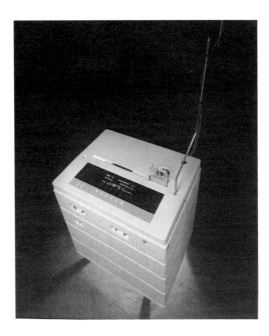

Figure 9-12. Photograph of the SLT Nd:YAG laser machine showing control panel and cartridge with the laser fiber.

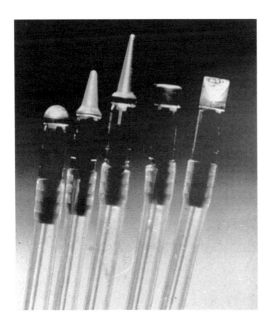

Figure 9-13. Photograph of the available Nd:YAG contact lasers with sapphire tips. The fibers are 2.5 mm in diameter and can be passed through a trochar into the joint. The tips can be used for cutting, ablation, or coagulation.

161

this, arthroscopy was performed on fresh frozen cadaveric knees. The second phase of our study involved three stages. First, articular-cartilage lesions were made with the laser and electrocautery on the femoral condyles of rabbits. Second, meniscectomies were performed, and regeneration at specific periods was compared for laser and electrocautery. Finally, meniscal repair was performed, and enhancement with low-level laser energy was evaluated.

The contact Nd:YAG laser with attachments, including a quartz-fiber delivery system and a sapphire tip, was used in our study. The first stage of the study involved seven fresh frozen canine cadaveric knees. Incisions were made on both medial and lateral femoral condyles and tibial plateaus (Fig. 9-14). In addition, single passes were made on the menisci. The wattage varied from 1 watt to 25 watts, and incisions were made using several different tips on the fiber. Specimens were subjected to histologic analysis, and depth of damage was measured. The depth of damage on both articular cartilage and meniscal tissue varied proportionately with power. At each wattage level, depth of damage was greater in meniscal tissue than in articular cartilage. This suggests that the laser preferentially cuts the meniscal tissue, which is an advantage clinically.

This preliminary study enabled us to select an appropriate wattage for subsequent research as well as for the clinical studies. The

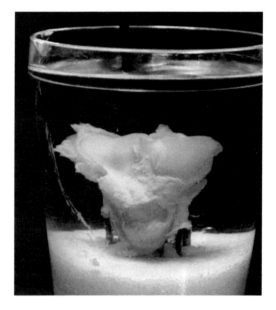

Figure 9-14. Photograph showing experimental arrangement for evaluation of Nd:YAG laser fiber with a contact tip. A cadaveric canine tibial plateau is mounted in the liquid medium. The laser fiber and contact tip are shown performing a menisectomy.

conical tip was selected because of its precise cutting, and the shorter version was used to facilitate the introduction of the tip into the joint through an arthroscopy portal.

Arthroscopy was performed on several fresh frozen human cadaveric knees (Col. Fig. 9-15). Following these procedures, appropriate fiber delivery systems were selected. Depending on the location of the lesion upon arthroscopy, one of three fiber delivery systems would be utilized (conization, oral, nasal). Tools adapted specifically for arthroscopic use are currently in development.

Although the laser eliminates the opening and closing problems encountered with current dissecting and cutting arthroscopy tools, the possibility of inadvertent contact with the articular surface must be addressed. This is partially overcome with the use of the foot pedal, which activates the laser only when the laser is situated in a safe cutting zone.

The second phase of our study included three stages. The first stage involved 24 adult New Zealand white rabbits undergoing bilateral knee arthrotomies.[9] In the first group of 12 rabbits, the Nd:YAG laser was used to make articular-cartilage lesions on the femoral condyles of one knee (Fig. 9-16). In the second group, an electrosurgical meniscectomy probe was used to make similar lesions on

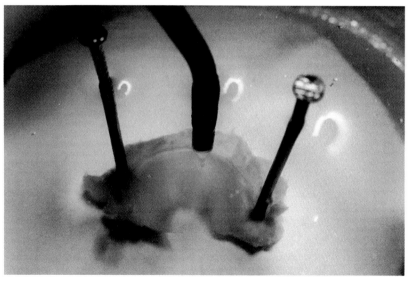

Figure 9 – 15. Photograph showing a cutting control tip being used to cut cadaveric human meniscus in a liquid medium.

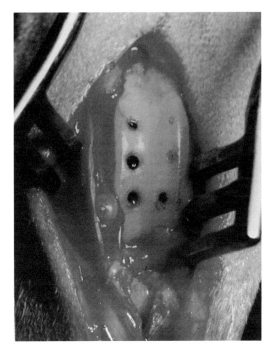

Figure 9-16. Photograph of laser menisectomy being performed in a rabbit knee. The contact cutting tip is shown excising the meniscus.

menisci (Fig. 9-17). In all 24 rabbits, similar lesions were made with a scalpel on the contralateral knee and served as controls in each case. The pulse duration of energy delivery for the laser and electrocautery was 1 second, with uniform pressure applied by a single surgeon. The wattage level varied from 10 watts to 30 watts for the laser and from 10 watts to 60 watts for the electrocautery. Scalpel lesions were made with a no.15 blade, and full-thickness incisions were attempted.

The rabbits were sacrificed at 1 day, 2 weeks, 6 weeks, and 12 weeks. The femoral condyles were harvested and, following fixation in 10% buffered formalin, were decalcified in 5% nitric acid solution in tap water. The articular surfaces were subjected to histologic analysis, which included hematoxylin–eosin and safranin O stains. Depth of damage was measured in all specimens, and areas of healing response were noted.

Vertical depth of damage created by the laser and electrocautery was comparable, with the laser penetrating subchondral bone at lower wattages. The healing response was quite different, however. Defects created by the laser showed a small margin of necrosis (less

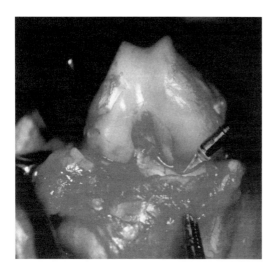

Figure 9-17. Photograph of a rabbit femoral condyle showing articular lesions that were created by the contact tips of the Nd:YAG laser.

than 0.2 mm). The laser incisions showed a vigorous healing response that was characterized at 6 weeks by chondrocyte proliferation, increased vascularity, and repair with hyaline cartilage followed by near-complete healing by 12 weeks. The elecltrocautery defects showed a significant lateral margin of necrosis (0.7 mm-1.8 mm) at increasing wattages that increased with time. By 12 weeks, there was little evidence of healing at wattage levels greater than 20 watts, and a limited response characterized by partial filling with tissue and fibrocartilage was seen at lower wattages.

The second stage of this study involved comparing the meniscal regeneration seen with laser, electrocautery, and scalpel.[10] Sixteen rabbits underwent bilateral knee arthrotomies. Bilateral medial and lateral meniscectomies were performed. Eight rabbits underwent medial laser meniscectomy on the left and medial electrocautery meniscectomy on the right. The second group of eight underwent lateral laser meniscectomy on the left and lateral electrocautery meniscectomy on the right. Scalpel meniscectomies (no.11 blade) were performed on the lateral menisci of the first group and the medial menisci of the second group. For the laser meniscectomies, a 1-second pulse was used with a wattage setting of 20 watts (average per rabbit was two pulses). Electrocautery was set at 20 watts (cut level), and the time of exposure was approximately 2 seconds.

Meniscectomies were performed in the middle third of the avascular portion of the menisci. Rabbits were sacrificed at 1 day, 2 weeks, and 12 weeks. The menisci were harvested and fixed in formalin. Following fixation, menisci were washed and sectioned. Histologic analysis with hematoxylin–eosin and safranin O stains was then performed. We have not yet completed this phase of the study.

The third phase of our study involved bilateral knee arthrotomies on eight rabbits to evaluate laser-enhanced meniscal repair. Scalpel incisions were made on the medial menisci of each rabbit. A 6-0 Prolene suture was used to repair the menisci. The left medial meniscus of each rabbit was exposed to laser energy at 10 watts for a 1-second pulse. A "frosted" laser scalpel tip rather than the conical tip used for cutting was used for this procedure. The frosted tip allows the dispersal of the energy from the entire surface area of the tip rather than at the endpoint only. We were able to place the tip within the incision, thereby effectively lasing the unexposed part of the scalpel defect. Full-thickness cuts were attempted with the scalpel in the midportion of the avascular zone of the meniscus.

Rabbits were sacrificed at 1 day, 1 week, 3 weeks, and 8 weeks. Menisci were dissected; following fixation in 10% buffered formalin, 6-0 Prolene sutures were removed, and menisci were then washed and sectioned. Histologic analysis included staining with hematoxylin and eosin and safranin O.

Results did not indicate that the laser energy at this wattage enhanced repair. No coagulum was visualized for any laser repairs at 1 day, 1 week, or 3 weeks. Rather, a band of acellularity was seen

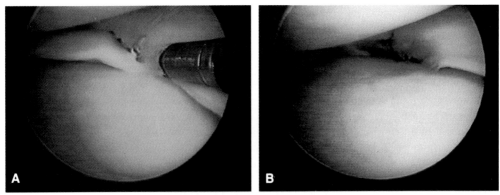

Figure 9–18. *A,* Intraoperative photograph through an arthroscope showing the Nd:YAG contact laser performing excision of the torn posterior horn of a medial semilunar cartilage. *B,* At the conclusion of the procedure, the torn portion of the meniscus has been cleanly excised.

along the incision where laser exposure occurred. This band of acel-lularity was not present in scalpel repairs. At 3 weeks, both groups looked histologically identical. It is possible that wattage level was too high in this instance. Attempts will be made with laser repair at lower wattage settings, and formation of coagulum will be evaluated. It would appear that laser-enhanced repair manifests itself only after the first week, as the band of acellularity seemed to increase from day 1 to week 1.

In addition to the favorable findings in the canine and rabbit studies, the contact Nd:YAG laser has also been used effectively in clinical studies at our institution.

We are currently conducting a clinical trial with the contact Nd:YAG laser for meniscectomies and to control bleeding in arthro-scopic acromioplasties. To date, we have done eight laser menisec-tomies and two arthroscopic acromioplasties using the contact Nd:YAG laser. We have been very satisfied with the early results. There have been no clinical complications, but one tip broke off inadvertently in the knee joint. This was retrieved without arthrotomy (Fig. 9-18).

From a biologic perspective the prospects for the future seem promising. At this time, we could consider the contact Nd:YAG laser superior to arthroscopic electrocautery; however, we do not recom-mend its widespread use until further basic-science investigation is completed and properly adapted arthroscopic instrumentation is fully tested.

REFERENCES

1. Whipple TL, Caspari RB, Meyers JF: Arthroscopic laser menisectomy in a gas medium. J Arthrosc Rel Surg 1, No. 1:2–7, 1985
2. Whipple TL, Caspari RB, Meyers JF: Arthroscopic menisectomy by CO_2 laser vaporization in a gas medium. Orthop Trans 6, No. 1:136, 1982
3. Fox JM, Ferkel RD, Del Pizzo A, et al: Electrosurgery in orthopaedics: Part II — applications to arthroscopy. Contemp Orthop 8, No. 2:37–44, 1984
4. Casscells SW: Arthroscopy: Diagnostic and Surgical Practice. Philadel-phia, Lea and Febiger, 1984
5. Rand JA, Gaffey TA: Effect of electrocautery on fresh human articular cartilage. J Arthrosc Rel Surg 1, No. 4:242–246, 1985
6. Snyder SJ: Letter to the editor. J Arthrosc Rel Surg 4, No. 2:147, 1988
7. Balduini FC, Peff TC, Torg JS: Application of electrothermal energy in arthroscopy. J Arthrosc Rel Surg 1, No. 4:259–263, 1985

8. Miller GK, Drennan DB, Maylahn DJ: The effect of technique on histology of arthroscopic partial meniscectomy with electrosurgery. J Arthrosc Rel Surg 3, No. 1:36–44, 1987
9. Miller DV, O'Brien SJ, Warren RF, et al: The use of the contact Nd:YAG laser in arthroscopic surgery: Effects on articular cartilage and meniscal tissue. Arthroscopy: The Journal of Arthroscopic and Related Surgery (Accepted for publication).
10. O'Brien SJ, Miller DV: The contact Nd:YAG laser: A new approach to arthroscopic surgery. Clinical Orthopaedics and Related Research (Accepted for publication).

Arthroscopic Surgery with the CO$_2$ Laser Wave Guide

Henry H. Sherk, Menachem M. Meller, and Anthony Rhodes

The CO$_2$ laser wave guide has only recently become available. It was described in Chapter 7 as a convenient and precise way of delivering CO$_2$ lasers deep into the femoral canal under direct visual control through a laparoscope. Basically, the wave guide is a hollow ceramic tube clad with stainless steel that can be snapped onto the end of the articulating arm of the laser. When the machine is activated the laser is conducted from the handpiece to the target. The beam is maximally focused at the end of the ceramic so that the spot size can be increased by moving the wave guide back away from the tissue or material to be vaporized. The metal cladding that protects the ceramic projects slightly beyond the tip of the ceramic permitting the operator to touch the target surface and even use the wave guide to probe the area of interest, thus providing some tactile feedback to the surgeon. A purge jet of CO$_2$ gas, which cools the wave guide, is directed through the wave guide at all times when the laser is being operated. The purge jet also protects the lenses of the laser from becoming fouled by retrograde passage of smoke and laser plume back up through the wave guide into the handpiece. The CO$_2$ gas purge jet has additional advantages of clearing the target surfaces of blood and debris, as well as preventing ignition of the laser plume. Wave guides were initially very expensive but they are now generally much cheaper and are, in fact, sold as disposable items to be used once and then discarded. Wave guides can also be fitted with reflective mirrors so that the beam does not have to be directed straight ahead during use. However, wave guides do cut down on the power of the laser and are brittle. During their use, therefore, the surgeon must increase the power setting slightly and be careful not to use the wave guide as a lever against resistant tissue. This might snap the ceramic core preventing efficient transmission of the laser beam.

The wave guide greatly facilitates laser arthroscopy. It can be inserted into a separate portal through a Stille's catheter or used in a "line of sight" fashion through an angled operating arthroscope. The angled mirror makes it adaptable and the laser beam can easily be directed anywhere in the joint. The procedure must, of course, be carried out with gas insufflation. The joint must first be distended with CO_2 at 60 mm of mercury through the arthroscope. We have found that this degree of insufflation permits the diagnostic arthroscopy to be performed. The Stille's catheter is then inserted and the wave guide is passed through the catheter into the joint. Loss of pressure in the joint is prevented by capping the Stille's catheter with a rubber stopper and passing the wave guide through the stopper. We have used wave guides with an outside diameter of 3.0 mm but smaller wave guides are available. It is important to maintain the purge jet pressure at a level higher than that of the insufflating CO_2 gas and the purge jet must have a continuous flow. This continuous inflow requires a venting outlet in the joint. This can be provided by inserting either an 18 gauge needle or a small Stille's catheter capped by a stopcock and opening the stopcock slightly to permit outflow of CO_2 gas. The surgeon should recognize that the purge jet inflow must be continuous and not activated by turning on the laser only because the laser plume will be blown back into the laser through the wave guide if the purge jet is not run continuously. The resultant clouding of the laser will cut down on the power of the laser and eventually occlude it altogether.

Once the surgeon has mastered the problems associated with the distension of a joint with a gas instead of saline, the use of the wave guide inside the joint is remarkably easy. The selection of a power setting and pulse modes have been addressed by Smith, Johansen, Vangsness, Sutter, and Marshall in an earlier section of this chapter. We have used a CO_2 laser wave guide with 15 watt power settings in

169

a superpulse mode to perform lateral releases, divide plicas, and cut meniscal tissue in 11 knees. In three knees with chondromalacia patellae we used a 5 to 10 watt superpulse laser to smooth off fibrillated articular cartilage on the lateral facet. Upon completion of the laser surgery in the joint, we irrigated the joints with saline and used a blunt probe to wipe away any carbonaceous material from the affected surfaces. One of the patients had a bloody effusion postoperatively. This was a 52-year-old woman with a bucket handle tear of the medial meniscus with degenerative arthritis. The laser was used to cut the posterior attachment of the bucket handle and the rest of the procedure was performed for the standard mechanical techniques. The cause of the effusion, therefore, is not clearly ascribable to the laser.

Arthroscopic surgery with a CO_2 laser wave guide has this year been approved by the Food and Drug Administration. Laser arthroscopy offers an attractive alternative to standard mechanical techniques but perhaps its ease of use and patient appeal may become adverse factors. Skilled arthroscopic surgeons must conduct controlled studies to establish the place of CO_2 laser arthroscopy. If it is used too widely and too soon, it may not find its proper place for a considerable period of time in the treatment of patients with joint pain. Other lasers may eventually prove superior. This is particularly true for the ultraviolet or excimer lasers, which are now in their earliest phases of development.

10

Foot Surgery with Lasers

Richard Smith
Anthony Rhodes
Henry H. Sherk

Foot surgery with lasers has been presented by some practitioners as a major advance in the treatment of foot disorders, and many patients appear to have accepted this as fact. We have therefore attempted to apply lasers to treatment of the foot in an effort to clarify the role of lasers in this type of surgery. We have found that lasers are, in fact, probably better than conventional means for cutaneous and toenail disorders, but at this time they seem to offer little benefit over mechanical devices for surgical treatment of disorders that involve the osseous elements of the foot.

As in other regions of the body, the laser may be used in three ways: as a light scalpel, as a cautery, and as a device to achieve tissue ablation. These uses roughly correspond to the CO_2, Nd:YAG, and argon lasers, respectively. The scalpel, osteotome, and oscillating saw are the instruments to which all surgeons are accustomed. They produce easy and precise cutting with tactile feedback to the surgeon. Although the CO_2 laser also provides easy and precise cutting, it is bulky, has a rigid articulating arm, and does not produce any tactile feedback. Because it works by vaporizing tissues, there is a risk of inducing thermal necrosis of surrounding tissues. The cut produced by the laser, however, is very precise, and because of its heat, it coagulates most small vessels. The laser incision is nearly bloodless, and this feature is an advantage over conventional techniques in foot surgery.

The drawbacks of the noncontact Nd:YAG are similar to those of the CO_2 laser. Because it uses a fiberoptic cable for carrying the light, it is not as cumbersome as the CO_2 laser, but it has a significantly deeper tissue penetration. This penetration has advantages and disadvantages. If more than 1 mm of tissue is to be ablated, then the Nd:YAG laser is preferable, but the full depth of the tissue effect may not be apparent for days after the surgery because sloughing occurs in the nonvaporized tissues. For this reason, it is sometimes advisable to use high power densities when using the Nd:YAG laser in order to fully vaporize the affected tissues. In addition, the char that is produced will somewhat limit the penetration of the radiation in the deeper tissues.

The sapphire-tipped touch technique of the Nd:YAG laser has not been widely used in foot surgery. The sapphire-tipped contact laser is basically a cautery, and it cuts more slowly than the noncontact Nd:YAG laser. Its benefits are tactile feedback and a very localized effect on only those tissues that are touched. The touch technique of the Nd:YAG laser offers no particular advantages over a scalpel, except the cauterizing effect.

The argon laser has only limited application because it is very selective in its absorption. The primary absorption of the laser in the body is by the porphyrin ring in the heme molecule. For this reason, however, vascular lesions such as hemangiomas are quite amenable to treatment with argon laser.

The skill of the surgeon is the factor that determines whether a laser is an improvement over the scalpel or electrocautery. The laser will cut or ablate the target tissues with minimal effect on the surrounding tissues, but power densities that are too high or too low and long exposure times increase the risk of unintended effects. The nontouch technique required by the laser necessitates some practice and technical adjustments. The surgeon loses the safety of tactile feedback and therefore risks unplanned cuts. There is also greater risk of injuring tissues deep to the target owing to the lack of a distinct endpoint, and there is some risk of overheating tissues surrounding the exposed area.

Current experience in foot surgery with lasers is based almost entirely on the CO_2 laser. This is because of the early introduction of this type of laser and the fact that the radiation of the CO_2 laser gives shallow tissue penetration and excellent vaporization. Care must be used in all laser applications to maintain the proper focus of the laser light. Under most circumstances, this means that the beam must be kept tightly focused to deliver the greatest power density. This will allow fastest cutting and minimum thermal damage to the surrounding tissue.

Maximum power density is achieved by keeping the laser tip at the distance of the focal length of the lens in the handpiece. The incidence of the beam should be kept perpendicular to the surface being cut. An oblique incidence will result in unequal tissue penetration owing to the variation in power density over the ellipsoid spot. In the region closest to the tip, the power density is greatest, and the density drops off rapidly in the further regions of the spot, resulting in uneven tissue penetration. Even penetration is especially important in applications requiring ablation of large areas of tissue.

ABLATIVE TECHNIQUES

The laser is an effective treatment modality for a number of common cutaneous and toenail diseases. In general, the patients remain ambulatory postoperatively, and the treatment usually can be accomplished in one visit.

Plantar Warts

The wart and thickened skin are first pared down to present a smooth surface. The Nd:YAG laser is applied to the wart and a small margin of uninvolved tissue. The tissues that are affected will assume a whitish discoloration. It is not necessary to use power densities that will vaporize the skin. The penetration of the Nd:YAG laser will be about 5 mm. Under most circumstances, this depth is ample for complete removal of the wart. The affected tissue will then slough off over the next few days and be replaced by normal epithelium. The advantage of the Nd:YAG laser is that the treated area has no bleeding and is relatively free of pain. The reason for this is the deep tissue penetration achieved by the laser without the need for skin incision or vaporization (Fig. 10-1).

The CO_2 laser produces its effect by vaporization only, and in this case, it is used more as a hyfrecator than a scalpel. After the usual prepping and draping, extraneous wart and hypertrophic skin are pared away to clarify the margins of the wart. A dermal curette is used to remove the majority of the lesion. The remaining bed of the wart may contain deep appendages of the wart and virus-infected cells, thus requiring further treatment using the CO_2 laser. Using a power density of approximately 5000 watts/cm², the bed of the wart is ablated. The operator should use slightly overlapping, even strokes of the laser. One should take care to prevent re-exposure of already

173

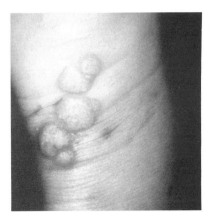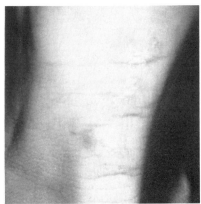

Figure 10–1. Plantar warts of the heel before and 2 months after treatment with the Nd:YAG laser. (Courtesy of Heraeus Laser Sonics.)

charred surfaces, as this will cause excessive heating of the underlying tissues. When the entire bed of the wart has been treated, the char should be wiped clean, and the procedure repeated until one can be reasonably sure that all infected tissue has been vaporized.

Postoperatively, the wound should be treated in the usual fashion with antibiotic ointment, dressing, and proper foot care. The patient's postoperative pain, swelling, and need for narcotics are often less when a laser is used for treatment.

Ingrown Toenails

Conventional treatment of ingrown toenails requires ablation of the nail bed by curettage with or without the use of a cauterizing substance such as phenol. Despite these measures, incomplete ablation of the ingrown nail does occur, often requiring an additional procedure. In our experience, the CO_2 laser has been more effective in achieving satisfactory matricectomy than conventional methods, and we have not noted regrowth of the nail in cases that we have treated with the laser. The laser may, in fact, be the best instrument for use in this type of case.

Partial Matricectomy

In partial matricectomy (Fig. 10-2), the toe is prepared for surgery by the use of a ring block using 1% lidocaine without epinephrine. A tourniquet can be applied to the base of the toe to ensure a bloodless field. Using a scalpel and elevator, the diseased portion of the nail is avulsed from the underlying matrix. Following this, ablation of the nail matrix may begin. The operator should use a power density of approximately 5000 watts/cm² and keep the beam perpendicular to the surface being treated. The matrix is ablated using strokes oriented transverse to the long axis of the toenail beginning proximally at the nail fold and proceeding distally. The speed of the strokes should be just fast enough to allow vaporization of the tissue but not so slow as to cause overheating. With vaporization, a char forms, and this will convert any further laser energy to heat, possibly resulting in damage to the underlying tissue. The strokes should overlap

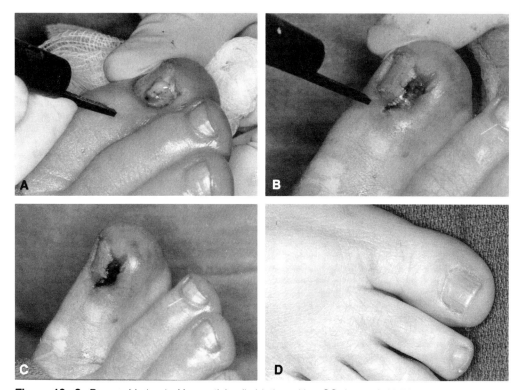

Figure 10–2. Paronychia treated by partial nail ablation with a CO_2 laser. *A*, Nail bed being incised. *B*, Nail bed being removed, and matrix being ablated with CO_2 laser at 15 watts of continuous power. *C*, Char seen after laser treatment. *D*, Three months after surgery.

175

slightly to avoid missing any matrix. The laser may be momentarily interrupted at the pause at the end of each stroke to prevent excessively deep penetration.

When the matrix in the nail bed has been ablated, attention may be turned to the nail fold. Special attention should be paid to the inferior surface of the fold because this is occasionally a site of incomplete ablation. When the entire matrix has been treated once, the char should be curetted free, and the entire procedure repeated to ensure complete ablation of the matrix.

The operator should excise by scalpel any hypertrophic skin that may have developed at the edge of the inwardly curving nail. The nail often imbeds deeply in the toe, and matrix may be imbedded deeply. Tissue overlying the imbedded edge should be excised to allow easy access for ablation. Following the matrix ablation, routine dressing and foot care should be instituted.

Complete Matricectomy

The technique for complete matricectomy (Fig. 10-3) is essentially the same as for partial matricectomy, except that a substantially larger area is being treated. The larger area results in greatly increased difficulty in achieving even ablation. Extra care must be taken in this circumstance to be sure that all the matrix has been ablated. Smooth, evenly spaced strokes of the laser will provide the best result.

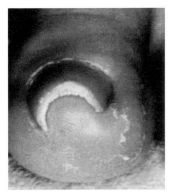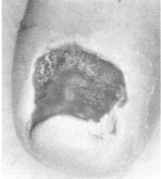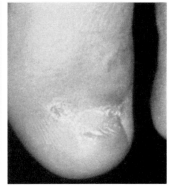

Figure 10-3. Complete matricectomy with CO_2 laser. (Courtesy of Heraeus Laser Sonics.)

ONYCHOMYCOSIS

The CO_2 laser has not been as effective as hoped in the treatment of fungal infections of the toenail. Both of the methods described below are effective, but neither is a significant improvement over standard techniques. The first technique involves avulsion of the toenail in a manner similar to the preparation for a complete matricectomy. After the avulsion, the hyperkeratotic nail bed is partially ablated using a power density of 5000 watts/cm². Unlike in matricectomy, the full thickness of matrix should not be ablated. Ablation that proceeds too deeply may result in defects in the regrown toenail. Postoperatively, the nail bed should be treated with topical antifungal ointment on a daily basis. It may also be necessary to treat the patient with a systemic antifungal medication such as griseofulvin.

The second method of treatment using the laser is to make multiple small perforations in the nail to provide topical antifungal medications access to the nail bed. The medication will then diffuse outward from the entry points to affect the entire nail bed. As the new nail grows out, it will be free from fungal infection.

SOFT-TISSUE DISSECTION

The value of the laser for soft-tissue dissection (Fig. 10-4) is the decreased inflammatory response of the tissue at the operative site. This effect is probably the direct result of sealing the small lymphatics and capillaries surrounding the incision. Several authors have reported an apparent reduction in postoperative pain in those patients who have had the soft-tissue dissection performed by laser. These represent individual case reports; there are no prospective studies at this time. Nevertheless, reduced blood loss and less postoperative pain are advantages in the use of the laser for soft-tissue dissection.[6]

OSTEOTOMY

We performed laser osteotomies and laser cheilectomies of the first metatarsal with satisfactory healing, but there was no obvious advantage to laser use in this regard. The laser osteotomy is more time consuming than the similar procedure using standard techniques.

We have concluded that the laser should not be used for osteotomy at this time. The lasers currently available cut bone only very slowly, with much thermal necrosis of surrounding osteocytes. The conventional mechanical methods of osteotomy are fast, effective, and well controlled. Using mechanical techniques, damage at the margins of the cutting is minimal and healing is rapid. The laser causes a wide zone of osteocyte necrosis and will prolong healing time. The excimer laser has been proposed as being effective for osteotomy, but there is no clinical experience with this application at the present time.

The use of the laser for bunionectomy does not require any special postoperative care. As stated above, some patients appear to have less postoperative pain than patients not treated with lasers.

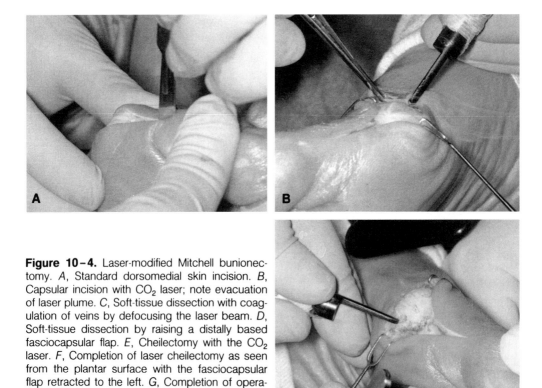

Figure 10–4. Laser-modified Mitchell bunionectomy. *A*, Standard dorsomedial skin incision. *B*, Capsular incision with CO_2 laser; note evacuation of laser plume. *C*, Soft-tissue dissection with coagulation of veins by defocusing the laser beam. *D*, Soft-tissue dissection by raising a distally based fasciocapsular flap. *E*, Cheilectomy with the CO_2 laser. *F*, Completion of laser cheilectomy as seen from the plantar surface with the fasciocapsular flap retracted to the left. *G*, Completion of operation, showing correction of deformity and skin closure.

SYNOVECTOMY

Synovectomy is a relatively limited and uncommon procedure about the foot and ankle. Laser synovectomy, however, can be performed with precision using the CO_2 laser. An excellent margin of safety is afforded by the strong absorption of the laser energy. The narrow region of ablation, however, may leave residual untreated synovium.

The Nd:YAG laser has a much deeper coagulation zone (up to 6 mm) and thus is better suited for synovial ablation. Additionally, the Nd:YAG laser has fiberoptic capability and can be used in a fluid medium. As previously noted, the tissue effect of the Nd:YAG laser is a zone of coagulated tissue that will slough over time, thus, the full

(Figure 10–4 continued)

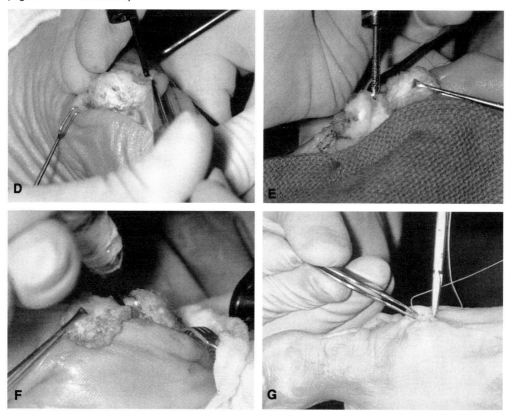

area of effect is not readily apparent at the time of surgery. A difficulty that the fluid arthroscopic medium imposes is the rapid conduction of heat away from the laser site. The coagulative effect of the laser is photochemical in part and not entirely dependent on raising the temperature at the laser site. The visually obvious effect, however, the wilting of the synovial fronds, is dependent on temperature. At low power densities, the heat is conducted away from the laser site before it reaches a sufficient temperature to cause frond wilting, thus, the surgeon may overexpose an area and cause undesirable damage to deep tissues. High power densities will induce visible tissue effects rapidly and will minimize the risk of overexposing the target. Clinical trials are presently being performed to determine the optimal power density and to fully delineate the postsynovectomy tissue effects.

CONCLUSIONS

The role of lasers in foot surgery is still unclear. Certainly both CO_2 and Nd:YAG lasers are effective in the treatment of disorders of the ectodermal appendages, such as plantar warts and toenail disorders, but they have not proved as preferable in other types of foot surgery. They do seem to result in less postoperative swelling, blood loss, and pain when used for soft-tissue dissection in bunion and toe surgery, but there are no scientific studies available to establish this point with certainty. An office laser of relatively low power for the treatment of cutaneous and toenail problems seems reasonable at this time, but it would seem appropriate only in high-volume clinics or practices that could justify the extra expense of a laser device. Higher powered and, thus, more expensive lasers that would be used in an operating-room setting are more adaptable for use in surgery that might include an osteotomy of a bone as small as a phalanx of a toe. Osteotomies of larger bones can be accomplished with lasers currently in use, but at this time mechanical means are still faster and easier. The excimer lasers and free-electron lasers may, however, make laser osteotomy preferable.

REFERENCES

1. Borovoy M: The treatment of verrucae vulgaris with carbon dioxide laser surgery. Clin Podiatr Med Surg. 4(4):799–807, 1987.

2. Borovoy M: Laser surgery in podiatric medicine: Present and future. Winter J Foot Surg 22(4):353–357, 1983.
3. Borovoy M: Laser safety in podiatry. J Foot Surg 24, No. 2:136–138, 1985.
4. Kaplan B: The carbon dioxide laser in podiatric medicine. Clin Podiatry, No. 2, 3:519–52, 1985.
5. McCarthy D: Therapeutic consideration in the treatment of pedal verrucae. Clin Podiatr Med Surg 2(1):433–448, 1986
6. Rothermel E: Carbon dioxide laser use for certain diseases of the toenails. Clin Podiatr Med Surg. 4(4):809–821, 1987.

11

Laser Discectomy

Henry H. Sherk
Anthony Rhodes

In the past decade, there has been great interest in minimizing the impact and magnitude of intervertebral disc surgery. Techniques of intradiscal chemonucleolysis with chymopapain or collagenase, microdiscectomy, and percutaneous discectomy have been offered as alternatives to the standard techniques of laminectomy (or laminotomy) and disc removal. Chymopapain injected into the intervertebral disc space to achieve chemonucleolysis (enzymatic removal of the disc) enjoyed considerable popularity in the early 1980s. Most patients, however, have back pain and paravertebral muscle spasm for several weeks postoperatively, and there is a small but frightening incidence of very severe complications associated with the procedure. As a result, fewer chemonucleolysis intradiscal injections are being done now than in 1983, when numerically the procedure was at its peak.[1] Microdiscectomy involves minimal dissection and morbidity, but some authors criticize the technique on the grounds that the very small field of vision limits the surgeon and prevents visualization of a broad enough surgical field. They point out that magnification made possible by the use of the microscope does not necessarily mean that a surgeon can see more if the operating field is so restricted.[6] Posterolateral percutaneous discectomy has also recently been described as a useful alternative to surgery done through a conventional laminectomy or laminotomy.[5] Only a few reports of patients treated with this technique are available, and there is no evidence that it is superior to the other methods described. The procedure has considerable appeal because of its limited morbidity. It is done under local anesthesia, usually on an outpatient basis, with a percutaneous insertion of either suction devices or a long-stemmed rougeur into the disc space. The proponents of the technique, however, note that it is not useful for an extruded disc fragment that has ruptured through the posterior longitudinal ligament into the spinal canal. Laser discectomy has been evaluated in a number of laboratories and in at least one clinical setting as an alternative to both conventional methods and the more recently described microdiscectomy and posterolateral percutaneous disc excision. In 1984, Gropper and colleagues reported that a CO_2 laser was effective in anterior discectomy in dogs and that it appeared as effective as mechanical techniques. It accomplished a more thorough disectomy in less time and was regarded as a potential time saver in this application. Since that time, Choy and coworkers[2] performed discal decompressions in experimental animals with the Nd:YAG laser. They noted that, in dogs, the Nd:YAG laser effectively decompressed discs and that there was no increase in morbidity in those animals treated with the laser as compared with those treated with conventional discectomy techniques. They expanded their study to include 12 patients. They injected 18-gauge needles into the disc space and threaded an Nd:YAG fiber through the needle into the space. With multiple short pulses, they were able to remove discal tissue and advance the fiber into the laser tract, decompressing the disc. the procedure was done under local anesthesia on an outpatient basis in these patients. Nine of the twelve patients experienced pain relief during the procedure, but five of the patients developed recurrent symptoms and required surgery. Since then, there have been additional reports on various types of lasers used in the laboratory setting.[4,8] One of the most interesting was that of Wolgin and associates,[7] who used an excimer laser through a fiber to ablate human intervertebral disc tissue. As might be expected, ablation rates varied with fluency (joules per square millimeter), in that the higher the fluency, the more rapid the penetration rate. The tissue developed a maximum temperature of 43.1°C at very high fluencies. Histologic evaluation showed no thermal damage to adjacent tissue after disc ablation with the excimer laser.

We have recently investigated the use of lasers in removing cervical intervertebral discs using 20-kg pigs as our experimental animals. We began by performing discectomies, decompressions, and nucleotomies on cadaveric cervical spines using both Nd:YAG laser fibers and a CO_2 laser waveguide fiber. Heretofore the CO_2 laser could only be used with a free beam; with a waveguide, however, the CO_2 laser can be delivered precisely to the intended target tissue at an exact power density. Both the Nd:YAG fiber and CO_2 waveguide permit transligamentous ablation of the intervertebral disc by permitting insertion of the laser into the disc space through a puncture wound in the anterior longitudinal ligament. We found that both types of lasers remove the tissue of the intervertebral disc very effectively when used in this manner. Well-localized ablation of the nucleus was achieved with 100 to 200 joules (watts per seconds), although more extensive tissue removal could be accomplished by more prolonged lasing with up to 800 joules.

To evaluate the possibility of thermal damage to the disc, bone, and cord, we placed thermocouples into the vertebral bodies, the vertebral end-plates, the posterior longitudinal ligaments, and the cervical cord using cadaveric specimens. We detected no rise in temperature in the cervical cord during laser disc ablation in the cadaveric specimens unless the laser beam penetrated the posterior longitudinal ligament and was directed against the cervical cord itself. When the laser was directed against the vertebral end-plates, there was a sustained local rise in temperature to 40 to 41°C, with several peak recordings up to 47°C, as recorded in the thermocouples in the end-plates. No rise in temperature was recorded in the vertebral bodies.

We also measured the intradiscal pressures before laser discectomy by inserting a needle into the center of the disc space and injecting saline through an Ivak manometer into the center of the disc. We recorded top pressures of 17 mm to 18 mm Hg in the normal discs.

We performed laser discectomies of the C4–5 intervertebral disc space using Nd:YAG and CO_2 lasers in living animals. The animals were anesthetized with intramuscular sodium pentothal and endotracheal nitrous oxide. The cervical spines were exposed anteriorly, and the disc-space pressure was recorded as described. The intradiscal pressures were the same in the living anesthetized animals as in the cadaveric specimens. We then inserted either the CO_2 waveguide or the Nd:YAG laser fiber through the anterior longitudinal ligament. The waveguide was inserted through a puncture wound slightly larger than the diameter of the guide to permit the laser plume to escape. The waveguide contained a coaxial CO_2 or nitrogen jet that forced the laser plume out of the disc space. We threaded a 2-mm Nd:YAG laser fiber through a large-bore needle with ample room available for the escape of any laser plume. We delivered 150 joules of laser energy into the disc space and then recorded the intradiscal pressure. After lasing in each instance, the pressure was recorded as zero. None of the animals manifested any ill effects from the procedure. They woke up promptly and walked about their cages without any evidence of neurologic impairment.

Four weeks postoperatively, the animals were euthanized with a sodium pentothal overdose. The cervical spines were removed, and the disc pressures were recorded. They were somewhat higher than those in the normal discs, probably because the disc spaces were replaced with dense, fibrous scar tissue. Roentgenograms showed some bridging by calcified tissue anteriorly in one animal, but the roentgenograms otherwise revealed normal-appearing disc spaces (Fig. 11-1A and B and Fig. 11-2).

Histologic evaluation showed dense scar tissue in the disc space with a marked alteration in the appearance of the normal nucleus pulposus (Fig. 11-3 and 11-4).

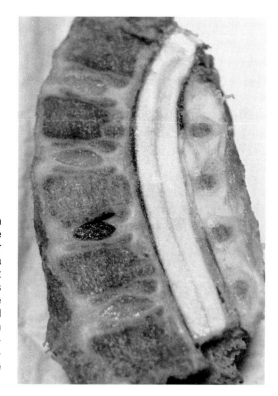

Figure 11-1. Photograph of sagittal section of porcine cervical spine 4 weeks after C4-5 disc ablation with a CO_2-laser wave guide (set at 20 watts in a continuous mode) for 60 seconds. The wave guide was inserted through a puncture wound in the anterior longitudinal ligament, and the disc was ablated by moving the wave guide.

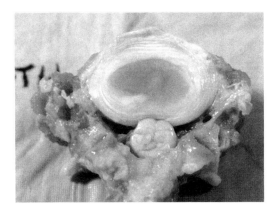

Figure 11-2. Photograph of transverse section of procine C3-4 disc 4 weeks after disc ablation with a Nd:YAG laser. The laser fiber was inserted into the middle of the disc space through a 16-gauge needle and 200 joules of energy were delivered to this area. The intradiscal pressure prior to the placement of the laser energy was 16 mm Hg as measured by injection of saline through an IVAK manometer. After lasering, the intradiscal pressure was zero.

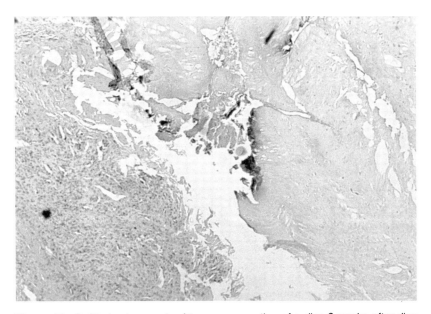

Figure 11-3. Photomicrograph of transverse section of a disc 6 weeks after disc ablation with the CO_2 laser. The disc has been replaced by fibrous tissue, and immature bone is noted in several areas throughout the disc space.

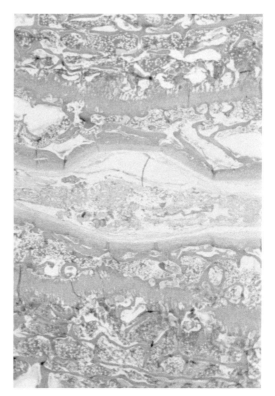

Figure 11–4.
Photomicrograph of sagittal section of porcine C4–5 cervical disc 4 weeks after treatment of disc with 200 joules of energy. The disc has been partially replaced by fibrous tissue.

CONCLUSION

We have concluded that a laser disc ablation with either a CO_2 laser waveguide or Nd:YAG fiber is safe without the likelihood of thermal injury to the cervical cord. Disc pressures fall to zero after delivery of only a small amount of focused laser energy into the disc space, and the disc is replaced by dense fibrous tissue in 4 weeks. There is the possibility that the disc space may be bridged by new bone if a longer period of time were allowed to elapse before the animals were euthanized.

REFERENCES

1. Agre K, Wilson RR, Brim M, et al: Chymodiactin post-marketing surveillance: Demographic and adverse experience data in 29,075 patients. Spine 9:479–485, 1984.
2. Choy DS, Case RB, Fielding W, et al: Letter: Percutaneous laser nucleolysis of lumbar disks. N Engl J Med, 317:771–772, 1987.
3. Gropper GR, Robertson JH, McClellan G: Comparative histological and radiographic effects of CO_2 laser versus standard surgical anterior discectomy in the dog. Neurosurgery 14:42–47, 1984.
4. Juri H, Ascher PW, Lillo J, et al: Lumbar disc nucleolysis by Nd:YAG laser radiation. An experimental comparative study (abstr). American Society for Laser Medicine and Surgery, Dallas, Texas. Lasers Surg Med 8:196, 1988.
5. Kambin P: Percutaneous posterolateral discectomy. Anatomy and mechanism. Clin Orthop Rel Res 223:145–154, 1987.
6. Microsurgical lumbar discectomy — another surgical gimmick? (editorial). Lancet 1, No. (8582):394–395, 1988.
7. Wolgin M, Finkenberg J, Papaioannou T, et al: Excimer laser ablation of human intervertebral disc (abstr). American Society for Laser Medicine and Surgery, Dallas, Texas. Lasers Surg Med 8:161–162, 1988.
8. Yanezama T, Matomura K, Atsumi K, et al: Intradiscal laser nucleotomy (abstr). American Society for Laser Medicine and Surgery. Dallas, Texas. Lasers Surg Med 8:205, 1988.

12

Cold Lasers

Gurvinder Uppal

Applications of lasers in medicine have diversified because of advancement in their accessibility, ease of use, and acceptance within the medical community. The conventional high-power lasers (in the power range of 10 watts to 100 watts) are discussed in other chapters. The low-power laser in the milliwatt range has fewer immediate applications in medicine. Its use is highly controversial. Some authors even consider it to be a gimmick.[2] Without making any biased judgement, current available knowledge on the low-power, or cold, laser is presented in this chapter.

In the United States, the infrared gallium–aluminum–arsenide laser, the visible helium–neon laser, and the argon laser are available as cold lasers. Since 1970, only the helium–neon laser has been approved for use by health-care providers in the United States.[1]

The helium–neon laser beam is used as the visible guiding beam for the invisible high-power lasers (*e.g.,* the CO_2 laser). The helium–neon laser beam penetrates tissue without divergence to 0.9 mm and only minimally to 10 mm to 15 mm. More than one half of its energy is absorbed by tissue located within 10 mm below the skin surface.[12] There are no reliable or uniformly accepted doses, power density, or time-effectual data available for the use of the helium–neon laser. The mechanism of efficacy of the helium–neon laser has yet to be resolved.

The helium–neon laser is used for biostimulation in aiding wound healing; for elevation of nerve-action potential in helping pain control; and for treatment of acute trigger points associated with nonspecific tendenopathies.

BIOSTIMULATION AND WOUND HEALING

The helium–neon laser delivers a light beam at a wavelength of approximately 630 nm with an average power output of 1.56 milliwatts. Typical treatments are done by lasering from 0.5 cm to 1.0 cm from the skin surface. The beam surface area is approximately 0.4 cm². Average treatment protocols require 300 seconds of laser treatment every other day until satisfactory results are achieved (Table 12-1).[5] Only 1.2 joules of energy are absorbed by tissue in each treatment, thus, no demonstrable elevation in tissue temperature is evident. At this energy level, it is recommended that one wear protective eyewear to prevent one from looking into the laser beam.

WOUND HEALING

Murine-model studies show helium–neon irradiated wounds have elevated tensile strengths. Elevations in tensile strength are evident 1 and 2 weeks postoperatively, but there is no difference at 8 weeks postoperatively when compared with nonirradiated wounds[4] (Fig. 12-1).[4] In vitro and in vivo models show elevated collagen production after helium–neon laser irradiation. Cell-culture models deficient in collagen production have shown accelerated collagen production after helium–neon laser irradiation. Clinical implications would be great if patients with impaired wound healing secondary to malnutrition, chronic infection, or steroid use would demonstrate accelerated wound healing. Studies from Budapest have shown decreases in pain and exudative discharge and eventual healing of chronically ulcerated and infected wounds sustained from coumarin-induced skin neurosis (Table 12-2).[7]

Table 12–1

Treatment Protocol for Wound Healing with Helium–Neon Laser*

Power: 1.56 milliwatts
Beam size: 0.385 cm²
Depth of penetration: 0.5 cm–1.0 cm from skin surface
Time/treatment: 300 sec

* Adapted from data in references 1 and 5.

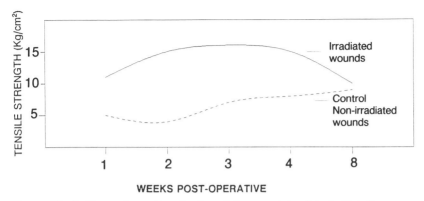

Figure 12–1. Comparison of tensile strength in wounds irradiated with helium-neon laser and nonirradiated wounds. (After Lyons R: Biostimulation of wound healing in vivo by a helium-neon laser. Ann Plast Surg 18:47–49, 1987.)

Swine-model studies from Rochester, Minnesota, showed no appreciable acceleration in wound closure, no increase in wound tensile strength, and no decrease in bacterial colonization after irradiation with a helium–neon laser. This study was done on animals with normal wound-healing properties.[1]

Mechanisms

Skin fibroblast cell cultures and murine studies show enhanced collagen accumulation after helium–neon laser irradiation. Radioactively labeled markers have demonstrated elevated type-1 and type-3 procollagen M-RNA levels at day 17 and day 28 in pig wounds after laser irradiation.[10] Incorporation of thymidine into cells, which is correlated with DNA synthesis and cell division, is unchanged

Table 12–2
Types of Wounds Either Cured or Improved with Helium–Neon Laser Irradiation*

Nonhealing skin ulcers after burns
Radionecrosis after radiation therapy
Diabetic lipodystrophy
Recurrent lymphangitis
Decubitus ulcers
Coumadin-induced skin necrosis

* Adapted from data in reference 7.

after laser irradiation.[6] Therefore, increased procollagen production cannot be accounted for by simple enhanced cell proliferation.

PAIN CONTROL

Pain control with conventionally accepted modalities of narcotic use, nonsteroid anti-inflammatory medication, and steroids is very variable in certain patients; therefore, it is difficult to get an objective quantification of pain.

Chinese physicians have used helium–neon laser irradiation at acupuncture points to relieve abdominal pain.[3] Scientific mechanisms for this are not understood. Several centers in the United States are treating chronic pain from osteoarthritis and tendenopathies using helium–neon laser irradiation. In patients with rheumatoid arthritis, cold laser irradiation resulted in pain resolution without any radiographic changes or changes in laboratory blood chemistry. Pain resolution seemed to be greater and of longer duration with lasers than with local heat-pack treatments.

Typical laser treatments involve 15 seconds to 20 seconds of continuous power at 1 milliwatt/cm^2 from 0.5 cm to 0.75 cm from the skin surface. This delivers 10 millijoules to 14 millijoules of energy. If there is a demonstrated initial response to three treatments, ten treatment sessions are typical (Table 12-3).

Clinical trials on patients with chronic pain of nonspecific etiology show equal decreases in discomfort in patients receiving actual helium–neon laser irradiation and those receiving placebo light treatment. Pain relief in both treatment groups lasted for 2 weeks, and there was a similar response to treatments in both men and women.[11]

Table 12-3
Treatment Protocol for Pain Control with Helium–Neon Laser*

Power: 1.56 milliwatts
Depth of penetration: 0.5 cm from skin surface
Time/treatment: 10 sec–15 sec
Number of treatments: 10–15 (after response to initial three sessions)

* Adapted from data in reference 12.

Mechanisms

Very few patients respond to helium – neon laser irradiation for pain control. It is hard to predict before treatment which patients will respond. This makes elucidation of the mechanism of lasers effect on pain control very difficult to support. Current studies in animal models have shown an elevation in 5-HIA levels after helium – neon laser irradiation. 5-HIA is a serotonin catabolic product. Serotonin is involved in the pain-control cascade; thus, its degradation may inhibit the sensation of pain without affecting the cause of the painful stimuli. Superficial radial nerve sensory latency is elevated with a decrease in conducting velocity after helium – neon laser irradiation.[8] This would also decrease or elevate the sensation of pain.

SUMMARY

Before helium – neon lasers receive widespread acceptance as the conventional treatment for aiding wound healing and pain control, more scientific studies need to be performed to shed light on its true mechanisms of action. Although relatively safe, the helium – neon laser, does have potential detrimental effects if one gazes into the beam with unprotected eyes. Therefore, its use should be limited to control trials by authorized personnel who are familiar with its use.

REFERENCES

1. Basford J: Comparison of cold quartz ultraviolet low-energy laser, and occlusion in wound healing in a swine model. Arch Phys Med Rehabil 67:151 – 154, 1985
2. Basford J: Low-energy laser treatment of pain and wounds: Hype, hope, or hokum. Mayo Clin Proc 61:671 – 675, 1986.
3. Hua T: Helium – neon laser irradiation of acupuncture points in treatment of 50 cases of acute appendicitis. J Tradit Chin Med 1:43 – 44, 1981.
4. Kana J: Effect of low-power density laser radiation on healing of open skin wounds in rats. Arch Surg 116:293 – 296, 1986.
5. Lyons R: Biostimulation of wound healing in vivo by a helium – neon laser. Ann Plast Surg 18:47 – 49, 1987.

195

6. Meyers A: Effects of low-watt helium–neon laser radiation on human lymphocyte cultures. Lasers Surg Med 6:540–542, 1988.
7. Mester E: Laser treatment of coumadin-skin necrosis. Acta Chir Acad Sci Hung 18:141–148, 1981.
8. Nissan M: Helium–neon laser irradiation delivered transcutaneously: Its effects on the sciatic nerve of rats. Lasers Surg Med 6:435–438, 1986.
9. Rochkind S: Electrophysiological effect of Helium–neon laser on normal and injured sciatic nerve in the rat. Acta neurochir 83:125–130, 1986.
10. Saperia D: Demonstration of elevated type I and type III procollagen mRNA levels in cutaneous wounds treated with helium–neon laser. Biochem Biophys Res Commun 138:1123–1128, 1986.
11. Siebert W: What is the efficacy of "soft" and "mid" lasers in therapy of tendinopathies? Arch Orthop Trauma Surg 106:358–363, 1987.
12. Snyder-Mackler L: Effect of helium–neon laser irradiation on peripheral sensory nerve latency. Phys Ther 68:223–225, 1988.

13

Future Applications of Lasers in Orthopaedics

Henry H. Sherk
Charles Kollmer
Menachem M. Meller

TREATMENT OF MUSCULOSKELETAL TUMORS WITH LASERS

Although lasers have been adapted to oncologic surgery and most other specialties (see Chapt. 4), they do not yet have a significant role in the treatment of musculoskeletal neoplasms. Their demonstrated effectiveness against pigmented noncalcified lesions in the treatment and palliation of gastrointestinal or genitourinary tumors, for example, would make one think that they would at least be useful in the treatment of synovial tumors and other extra-osseous, noncalcified tumors in extremities such as rhabdomyomas or soft-tissue sarcomas. Tumors in bone pose special problems, but even the commonly available CO_2 and Nd:YAG lasers might have usefulness in the treatment of bone tumors if the technology were developed. Nevertheless, the lack of any published information on the clinical effectiveness of lasers in musculoskeletal oncology certainly indicates that their use in the treatment of tumors of the extremities and axial skeleton will require a great deal of effort if they are to be used successfully in the future.

An obvious advantage to laser use in oncologic surgery is the effect lasers have on tissue surrounding a tumor. The small vessels, capillaries, and lymphatics are sealed by the laser, thus lessening the possibility of tumor spread when such lesions are excised. In the resection of a tumor within a compartment or in the radical resection of an entire compartment, this property of the laser might be of potential benefit. If an intralesional resection is possible, the laser can also be used to ablate the tumor bed.

Although our own experience is limited, we did find the laser useful in villonodular synovial lesions from joints. Figures 13-1, 13-2, and 13-3 (Col. Figs 13-2 and 13-3) illustrate a case in which a Nd:YAG laser set at 30 watts in continuous-wave mode ablated the base of the synovial lesion and smoothed out the tissue lining the inferior capsule. Approximately 3000 joules were used in this application. To date, there has been no evidence or recurrence in this patient (follow-up at 6 months). We have also used the laser to cauterize the bed of enchondromas, nonossifying fibromas, and low-grade giant cell tumors. These reports, of course, are anecdotal, and the laser was used as an adjunct to conventional curettage and bone grafting. Nonetheless, the laser appeared convenient and effective and seemed to offer some promise in the treatment of skeletal lesions.

Photodynamic therapy, which was described briefly in Chapter 4, entails the use of lasers in an uniquely effective, albeit indirect, method.[1-8] The treatment is based on the observation that tumor tissue takes up hematoporphyrin following systemic administration. Initially, this phenomenon was useful in diagnosis because the tumor tissue labeled with the hematoporphyrin could be visualized by fluorescence when it was exposed to ultraviolet light.[5] It has also been learned that the hematoporphyrins very strongly absorb laser light in the red violet band around 400 nm[1]. Upon absorbing light in

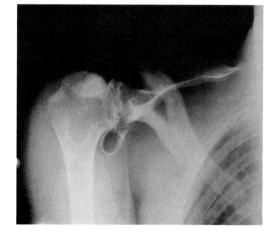

Figure 13–1. Preoperative roentgenogram of the right shoulder of a 27-year-old man showing a pigmented villonodular synovitis. The diagnosis was established by arthroscopy and biopsy.

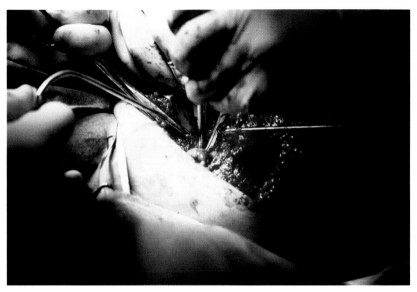

Figure 13–2. Intraoperative photograph showing the pigmented villonodular synovitis prior to ablation with the laser.

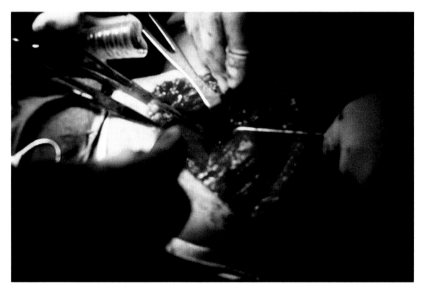

Figure 13–3. Intraoperative photograph showing the shoulder after ablation of the lesion with a Nd:YAG laser.

this band, the hematoporphyrin photosensitizer undergoes photo-chemical reactions involving the formation of an excited singlet state of oxygen from the excited triplet state.[4] This energy-transfer process produces irreversible oxidation of organic molecules with destruction of the sensitized cell labeled with the hematoporphyrin. The death of the tumor cell, which had absorbed the photosensitizing agent, is the basis for the development of this field of tumor therapy.

Photodynamic therapy thus involves preferential absorption of the photosensitizing dye by tumor tissue as opposed to normal surrounding tissue.[6] Most of the research done in this area has involved hematoporphyrin or its derivatives, such as photophrin I (dihemato-porphyrin ether) and photophrin II (dihematoporphyrin ester).[6,7] Other agents, such as chlorophylls, bacterchlorophylls, purpurines, and chlorins, are under development.[2,3] Because many of the tumors encountered in orthopaedics are relatively avascular, there is relatively little chance for these photosensitizing agents to be selectively absorbed, and new combinations of photosensitizing agent and laser wavelength may have to be discovered before this branch of treatment has wide applicability in musculoskeletal oncology. Photodynamic therapy has yielded encouraging results, however, in the treatment of solid tumors of the bronchus, esophagus, head and neck, skin, and eye, and its application to musculoskeletal lesions may lie in the future.

Interstitial hyperthermia is a technique that appears to enhance photodymanic therapy. It entails the introduction of a laser fiber into a tumor mass, which raises the temperature of the neoplastic tissue locally. The rise in temperature within the tumor tissue causes an increase in the metabolism of the tumor cells. Although the increased metabolic responses may have a lethal effect on the cell itself, the lethal effect is greatly enhanced when the interstitial therapy is combined with photodynamic therapy.[8]

LASER DIAGNOSTICS

Laser Doppler flowmetry (LDF) is a noninvasive technique for measuring tissue microcirculation and red-blood-cell flow.[6,14] During the past decade, it has been utilized to monitor free-flap viability,[11,13] predict flap necrosis[4,7,16] evaluate blood flow in bone,[8,17,18] and assess tissue blood flow in occlusive vascular diseases such as Raynaud's disease[3] and arteriosclerosis.[1,9,10,12] Stern[15] investigated the physics of LDF in 1978. He observed that the coherent light of a milliwatt helium–neon laser beam was scattered from a complex medium that was in internal motion. The spectrum of the beam was broadened by the Doppler effect. He used an electronic spectrum analyzer to evaluate the band width of the reflected beam and used this information to measure red-blood-cell flux in tissues.

Laser Doppler flowmetry depends on the Doppler principle, in which the laser light that strikes a moving object will undergo a shift in frequency proportional to the velocity of the moving object. Because the light reflected from the moving red blood cells in tissues undergoes multiple scattering, LDF requires that the Doppler shifted beam be compared with the "reference beam" being reflected from stationary elements in the tissue being evaluated. The instrument includes a 2-milliwatt helium–neon laser directed through the head of a probe directly onto the tissue. The laser light penetrates the tissue to a depth of 0.5 mm to 1.0 mm, and the red blood cells passing through this volume of tissue strike the light and reflect it back into the instrument, where the Doppler shift is evaluated electronically.

Laser Doppler flowmetry and modified photoplethosmography are the only noninvasive methods of continuously monitoring circulation in tissues at this time. Subjective assessments, such as evaluation of tissue color, dermal bleeding, and capillary refill time, are occasionally inaccurate, and transcutaneous CO_2 measurements are invasive and potentially damaging to tissues.[19] Fluorescein evaluation of tissue blood flow has been criticized as possibly underestimating flap viability.[7] Laser Dopplar flowmetry appears to be accurate and efficient, and it correlates well with other tests now used in the determination of soft-tissue viability as determined by assessment of red-blood-cell flow. Not all investigators, however, have recognized LDF as an important clinical methodology in the evaluation of tissue blood flow, and at least one investigator has termed LDF as "superfluous" and "of limited value."[11] Judging from the recent literature, however, most authors do consider LDF an important new technology in the assessment of the viability of soft tissues.

Swiontowski and coworkers,[17,18] reported on the use of LDF in determinations of red-blood-cell flux in bone. They noted the obvious appeal of such a technique because currently assessment of blood flow in bone requires biopsy or insertion of a sensor into the bone. These invasive procedures alter the local conditions of the tissue and render hydrogen washout, 133 Xenon washout, microsphere estimation, and indicator fractionation difficult to use clinically. Bone scintigraphy and magnetic resonance imaging, provide important preoperative information, but there is a need for an accurate, easy-to-use system for making determinations of bone viability intraoperatively. Laser Doppler flowmetry may become useful in this regard in the future.

Sophisticated laser-based diagnostics are continuously being developed.[2,5] Nephelometry, for example, is a measurement of the cloudiness of solutions. Analysis of various fluids for a particular content or light-transmission characteristics is possible with this technique. Several authors have reported, that laser nephelometry is a simple and effective method for evaluation of rheumatoid synovial fluid. Lasers are also useful in the development of temperature response curves for various materials and in the detection of extremely small changes in material properties such as reflectance and weight.

These technologic developments have considerable importance for orthopaedic surgeons because they may provide for quick, inexpensive, and extremely accurate measurements of clinical information that heretofore has been difficult to obtain. For the time being, the advancement of the technology appears to have outstripped the clinician's ability to apply it, but the future of these diagnostic modalities appears intriguing.

REFERENCES

Treatment of Musculoskeletal Tumors with Lasers

1. Dougherty TJ, Grindley GB, Fiel B, et al: Photoradiation therapy II: Cure of animal tumors with hematoporphyrin and light. J Natl Cancer Inst 55L115–119, 1975
2. Gomer CJ, Ferrario A, Hayashi N, et al: Molecular, cellular, and tissue responses following photodynamic therapy. Lasers Surg Med 8:450–463, 1988
3. Getenby RA, Hammond ND, Brown DQ: Tumor therapy with hematoporphyrin derivative and lasers with a percutaneous fiberoptic technique. Radiology 163:167–171, 1987
4. Henderson BW, Miller AC: Effects of scavengers of reactive oxygen and radical species on cell survival following photodynamic treatment in vitro: Comparison to ionizing radiation. Radiat Res 108:196–205, 1986
5. Lipson RL, Grey MJ, Baldes EJ: Hematoporphyrin derivative for detection and management of cancer. Cancer 20:2255–2257, 1967

6. Moon J, Christensen T, Sommers S: The main photosensitizing components of HpD. Cancer Letter 15:161–166, 1982
7. Moon J, Johanssen JF, Christensen T, et al: Porphyrin-sensitized photoinactivation of human cells in vitro. Am J Pathol 109:184–188, 1982
8. Waldow SM, Morrison PR, Grosweiner LI: Nd:YAG laser-induced hyperthermia in a mouse tumor model. Lasers Surg Med 8:510–515, 1988
9. Weishaupt, KR, Gomer CJ, Dougherty TJ: Identification of singlet oxygen as the cytotoxic agent in photoinactivation of a murine tumor. Cancer Res 36:23–26, 1976

Laser Diagnostics

1. Cochrane T, et al: Laser Doppler flowmetry in the assessment of peripheral vascular disorders. A preliminary evaluation. Clin Phys Physiol Meas 7:31–42, 1986
2. Cohn JR, Buckley CE 3rd Connell CD: Simplified screening for immune complexes by laser nephelometry of ultracentrifuge serum. Diagn Immunol 2, No.(3):175–180, 1984
3. Engelhart M, et al: Raynauds phenomenon: Blood supply to the fingers during indirect cooling, evaluated by laser Doppler flowmetry. Clin Physiol 6:481–488, 1986
4. Fischer JC, Pailser, PM, Shaw, WW: Laser Doppler flowmeter measurements of skin perfusion changes associated with arterial and venous compromise in the cutaneous island flap. Microsurgery 6:238–243, 1985
5. Geissler N, Kemper A, Krapf E, et al: Demonstration and differentiation of circulating immune complexes in chronic inflammatory rheumatic diseases using a semiautomatic PEG-precipitation laser nephelometer test. Z Rheumatol 44:57–63, 1985
6. Haumschild DJ: An overview of laser Doppler flowmetry. Biomed Sci Instrum 22:35–40, 1986
7. Heden P, Jurell G, Aruander C: Prediction of skin-flap necrosis: A comparative study between laser Doppler flowmetry and the fluorescein test in a rat model. Ann Plast Surg 17:485–488, 1986
8. Hellein S, Jacobson LA, Nilsson GE, et al: Measurement of microvascular blood flow in cancellous bone using laser Doppler flowmetry and 133Xe clearance. Int J Oral Surg 12:165–168, 1983
9. Koranfilian RG, et al: The value of laser Doppler velocimetry and transcutaneous oxygen tension determination in predicting healing of ischemic forefoot ulcerations and amputations in diabetic and non-diabetic patients. J Vas Surg 4:511–516, 1986
10. Leonardo G, Arpaia MR, Del Guercio R: A new method for the quantitative assessment of arterial insufficiency of the limbs: Cutaneous post-ischemic hyperemia test by laser Doppler. Angiology 38:378–385, 1987

11. Lerche A, Paaske WP: Laser Doppler examination of microvascular reactivity. Surg Gynecol Obstet 163:410–414, 1986

12. Masten FA, Wyss CR, Robertson CL, et al: The relationship of transcutaneous PO_2 and laser Doppler measurements in a human model of local arterial insufficiency. Surg Gynecol Obstet 159:418–422, 1984

13. Powers EW, Frazer WF: Laser Doppler measurements of blood flow in microcirculation. Plast Reconstr Surg 61:250–255, 1978

14. Smits GJ et al: Evaluation of laser Doppler flowmetry as a measure of tissue blood flow. J Appl Physiol 61:666–672, 1986

15. Stern MD: In vivo evaluation of microcirculation by coherent light scattering. Nature 254:56–58, 1975

16. Svensson H et al: Laser Doppler flowmetry and laser photometry for monitoring free flaps. Scand J Plast Reconstr Surg 19:245–249, 1985

17. Swiontkowski MF, Ganz R, Schlegel V, et al: Laser Doppler flowmetry for clinical evaluation of femoral head osteonecrosis: Preliminary experience. Clin Orthop Rel Res 218:181–185, 1987

18. Swiontkowski MF, Tepic S, Perren SM, et al: Laser Doppler flowmetry for bone blood flow measurement: Correlation with microsphere estimates and evaluation of intracapsular pressure on femoral head blood flow. J Orthop Res 4:362, 1986

19. Valdez-Cruz LM, Yoganathan AP, Tamura T, et al: Studies in vitro of the relationship between ultrasound and laser Doppler velocimetry and applicability to the simplified berinoulli relationship. Circulation 73:300–308, 1986

14

Excimer Lasers

Menachem M. Meller

An excimer (excited dimer) is a metastable dimer molecule formed by a transient combination of an atom of a noble gas with an atom of halogen. Due to the nanosecond decay of the molecule, this laser operates in a pulsed mode. The emitted radiation is in the ultraviolet range (106 nm–400 nm) and has excellent absorption in organic polymers and biologic proteins. Laser pumping is by means of an electrical discharge, the frequency of which determines the pulsing frequency. The five commonly used excimer gases are argon fluoride, krypton chloride, krypton fluoride, xenon chloride, and xenon fluoride, with wavelengths of 193 nm, 222 nm, 249 nm, 308 nm, and 350 nm, respectively. The lasing chamber is filled with 0.06% halogen and 0.15% noble gas, and the remainder is diluent. The potential health hazards of the laser are the toxic gases of the lasing medium, the radio frequency emitted by the pumping source, and the potential mutagenicity at the DNA absorption peak of 248 nm. Innovations in laser design have minimized the first two effects. Recent studies of anaplastic transformation following ultraviolet exposure indicate that the concern is not as great as was once believed.[5,22]

Much of the literature dealing with ultraviolet lasers and biologic tissues comes from the ophthalmology, cardiovascular, and dermatologic literature. The process of ablative photodecomposition deals with the nonthermal disruption of chemical bonds. The basic premise is that proteins contain chromophores, which can absorb quanta of a given wavelength and cause cleavage of specific peptide bonds without any thermal damage. The dynamics of this process have been studied by chemical kinetics and the reaction products,[4] laser-based high-speed photography,[16] and ultrastructural studies using histology and scanning electron microscopy.[1–3,7–11,13,14,17] Wound-healing studies have been done as well. Regardless of the tissue being cut, ultrastructural studies revealed a remarkably precise and accurate excimer cut (Figs. 14–1 to 14–4). The vapor-phase photodecomposition products, however, are indistinguishable from continuous-wave laser irradiation or flame torching of cardiovascular tissues. In both instances, the products contained methane, acetylene, ethylene, ethane, propylene, allene propylene, propane, and butane.[4] As Morelli and coworkers[12] indicate, it may be the means of energy delivery and not the wavelength itself that is responsible for the unique type of tissue removal.

The parameters that can be varied for excimer lasers are wavelength, fluence, frequency, pulse duration, peak power, power per pulse, average power, and spot size. Wavelength is a parameter that varies with the lasing medium. Fluence, defined as the energy per pulse per unit area equals the energy per pulse per spot size. This value can be varied from a maximum by optical attenuators. Pulse duration and peak power are often determined by the laser design, especially for industrial-type lasers. One is therefore left with only one true independent variable — namely, the pulse frequency and thereby the average power. It is crucial, however, to specify the preceding parameters correctly in order to obtain satisfactory results.

As far as tissue effects are concerned, it has been shown that over limited ranges, spot size does not affect etch depth at constant fluence[20] and is identical to the ablated area.[12] There are conflicting reports as to whether pulse duration has any effect on etch depth. There is uniform agreement, however, that ablation rates and etch per pulse increase monotonically with fluence. Increasing the

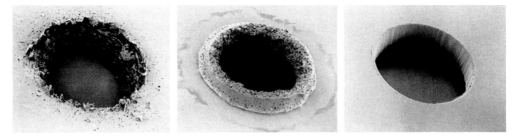

Figure 14-1. Comparison of 300-μm diameter holes drilled in a 75-μm thick polyimide sheet using three common types of lasers. The SEM photograph on the left-hand side corresponds to a pulsed Q-switched Nd:YAG laser operating at 1.06 μm. The middle photograph corresponds to a fast axial flow CO_2 laser operating in a pulsed mode. The right-hand photograph corresponds to an excimer laser at 248 nm. Note the high degree of precision in the excimer case, and the absence of any damage to the surrounding material. (Courtesy of Lumonics Inc.)

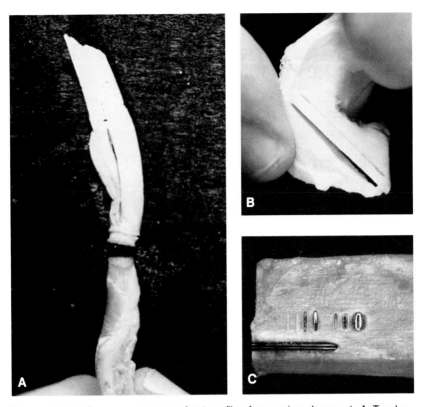

Figure 14–2. Gross appearance of cut profile of an excimer-laser cut. *A*, Tendon. *B*, Meniscus. *C*, Bone. Operating conditions were xenon-fluoride of wavelength 308 nm; a power density of 2 milliwatts/cm²; and a pulse duration of 20 nsec.

fluence or energy per pulse and increasing the pulse frequency have been reported to increase the thermal damaged zone.[12]

A typical ultraviolet laser pulse contains about 170 millijoules, a 10-nsec (nanosecond-billionth of a second) duration, and a fluence of 68 millijoules/cm². As a matter of interest, the peak power of such a pulse reaches 10^6 watts, the sustained power of a large electric generator. The laser's average power would be 25.5 watts at a pulse frequency of 150 hertz. The power density would be 10.2 watts/cm² far below the 50,000 watts/m² used with a CO_2 laser. The cross section of such a beam is 2.5 cm² or about 8333 times the focused area of a CO_2 beam. For an excimer laser, this is a respectable amount of power. The broad beam allows surfaces to be ablated by

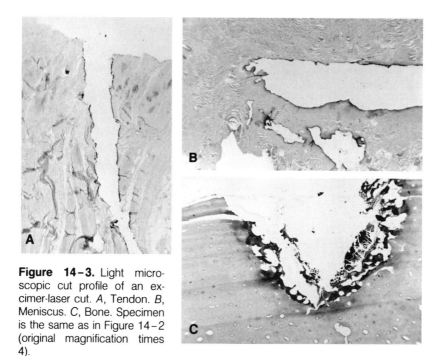

Figure 14-3. Light microscopic cut profile of an excimer-laser cut. *A*, Tendon. *B*, Meniscus. *C*, Bone. Specimen is the same as in Figure 14-2 (original magnification times 4).

etching rather than carving, as done by a CO_2 laser. Although this may be an advantage for material processing for tissues, an appropriate pinhole or slot mask can create the desired drill hole or tissue cut.

When a beam with the preceding characteristics is incident to a tissue surface, there is a minimum fluence below which no visible effects occur. This quantity, termed the *threshold fluence,* has been explained as that energy required to exceed competing thermal and nonthermal energy losses. Typically, there is a delay of 5 nsec to 10 nsec before any observable changes occur in the tissues as measured by the stress pulse. This delay may be the time necessary to initiate ablation and to accelerate the ablated particles into the gas plume. Puliafito and colleagues[16] have demonstrated using high-speed laser-based photography that a plume is formed at about 0.5 μsec and is generally complete by 5 μsec to 15 μsec for a 193-nm pulse. The ablation products leave at supersonic velocities and decelerate rapidly. At an operating frequency of 100 hertz, the time interval between pulses is $10^4\ \mu$sec $= 10^7$ nsec, so that a laser plume lasting 150 μsec is unlikely to cause thermal damage.

208

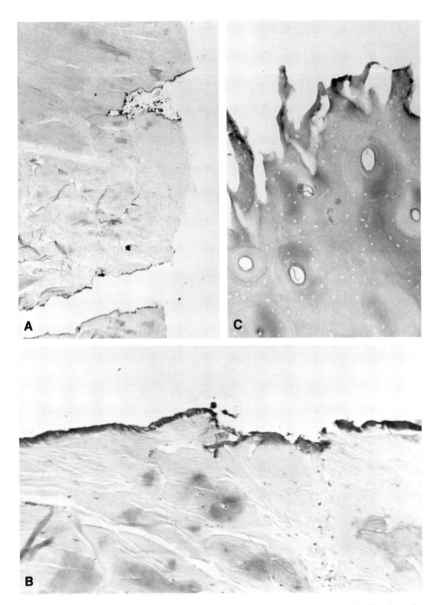

Figure 14–4. Light microscopic cut profile of an excimer-laser cut. *A*, Tendon. *B*, meniscus. *C*, Bone. Specimen is the same as in Figure 14–2 (original magnification ×10).

The cut properties of tissues differ nonpredictably for various wavelengths. Nonevicz and coworkers[14] measured the ablation rate of ocular lens and the ablation threshold and found them to be highest at the midrange wavelength of 248 nm. Absorbance was measured with a spectrophotometer and was highest at the shortest wavelength. This high absorption, or, conversely, decreased penetration depth, partly explains the best edge definition found with 193-nm beams. At this wavelength, the penetration depth for corneas is about 7 μm with an ablation depth per pulse of 1 μm to 4 μm depending on the fluence. The thermal-diffusion length for a pulse duration of 20 nsec is about 0.1 μm. We have a process whereby micron-thick tissue sections can be rapidly ablated by using high repetition rates — an ideal compromise between speed and control.

Nearly all the ultrastructural studies reveal a very narrow zone adjacent to the ablation crater. This zone has been referred to as either basophilic stipling, pseudomembrane, or thermal necrosis. This zone was seen to be greatest at wavelength of 248 nm by increased pulse frequency and fluence. An explanation for this phenomenon was given by Morelli and colleagues with the thermal relaxation time. Thermal relaxation time is defined as that time required for the tissue to cool to one half the original value (thermal relaxation time = penetration depth^2 [reciprocal of absorbance]/twice the thermal diffusivity in water). With a penetration depth of 10 μm at 193-μm wavelength and a thermal relaxation time of 238 μsec, one would have to pulse at rates greater than 2.6×10^3 sec^{-1} to create thermal injury. For a laser wavelength of 248 nm and a penetration depth of 100 μm, thermal relaxation time is 38 msec, and one just needs to exceed 26 pulses to create thermal injury. In practice, thermal relaxation time is difficult to measure because conventional thermocouples respond at best in the millisecond range. Practically, one can therefore think of the precision of the excimer cut being attributed to a purely nonthermal mechanism accompanied by thermal damage, or else the entire mechanism may be thermomechanical.

For a practicing orthopaedist, the exact mechanism of action of excimer lasers is immaterial. Of utmost importance, however, is a clean cut, ease of use, minimal thermal damage, and good wound healing. The laser must be sufficiently powerful and safe and have an easy means of delivery to the tissues. Preliminary evidence indicates that the lowest ultraviolet wavelength provides the best edge definition without thermal damage. Unfortunately, technical limitations make it difficult to make a flexible fiber delivery system for less than 200 nm, especially at high power. The lack of such a delivery system would make arthroscopic surgery difficult.

Also of concern to the practitioner is having an expensive piece of equipment designated as being necessary to delivery the standard of care. Even more disturbing would be the thought of having such a piece of equipment rendered obsolete, requiring replacement in a short period. From a review of the literature, it appears that there are only two possibilities of lasers adequate to cut bone and soft tissue (*i.e.,* the free-electron laser and tunable dye laser). Neither of these can conceivably be built at an affordable price with adequate power in the near future. Excimer lasers, therefore, may be a replacement for the surgical scalpel in the near future.

REFERENCES

1. Aron R, Boerner CF, Bath P, et al: Corneal wound healing after excimer laser keratotomy in a human eye. Am J Ophthalmol 103:454–464, 1987
2. Bath PE, Mueller G, Apple DJ, et al: Excimer laser lens ablation. Arch Ophthalmol 105, No. 9:1164–1165, 1987
3. Berlin MS, Rajacich G, Duffy M, et al: Excimer laser photoablation in glaucome filtering surgery. Am J Ophthalmol 103, No. 5:713–714, 1987
4. Clarke RH, Isner JM, Donaldson RF, et al: Gas chromatographic-light microscopic correlative analysis of excimer laser photoablation of cardiovascular tissues: Evidence for a thermal mechanism. Circ Res 60, No. 3:429–437, 1987
5. Green H, Boll J, Parrish JA, et al: Cytotoxicity and mutagenicity of low intensity, 248- and 193-nm excimer laser radiation in mammalian cells. Cancer Res 47, No. 2:410–413, 1987
6. Hanna K, Chastang JC, Pouliquen Y, et al: A rotating slit delivery system for excimer laser refractive keratoplasty. Am J Ophthalmol 103:474, 1987
7. Jacques SL, McAuliffe JD, Blank IH, et al: Controlled removal of human stratum corneum by pulsed laser. J Invest Dermatol 88, No. 1:88–93, 1987
8. Kerr-Muir MG, Trokel SL, Marshall J, et al: Ultrastructural comparison of conventional surgical and argon fluoride excimer laser keratectomy. Am J Ophthalmol 103:448–453, 1987
9. Lane RJ, Wynee JJ, Geronemus RG: Ultraviolet laser ablation of skin: Healing studies and a thermal model. Lasers Surg Med 6, No. 9:504–513, 1987
10. Lieurance RC, Patel AC, Wan WL, et al: Excimer laser cut lenticules for epikeratophakia. Am J Ophthalmol 103:475–476, 1987

11. McDonald MB, Beuerman R, Falzoni W: Refractive surgery with the excimer laser. Am J Ophthalmol 103:469, 1987

12. Morelli J, Kibbi AG, Farinelli W, et al: Ultraviolet excimer laser ablation: The effect of wavelength and repetition rate on in vivo guinea pig skin. J Invest Dermatol 88(6):769–773, 1987

13. Murphy-Chutorian D, Selzer PM, Kosek J, et al: The interaction between excimer laser energy and vascular tissue. Am Heart J 112(4):739–745, 1986

14. Nanevicz TM, Prince MR, Gawande AA, et al: Excimer laser ablation of the lens. Arch Ophthalmol 104(12):1825–1829, 1986

15. Prodouz KN, Fratantoni JC, Boone EJ, et al: Use of laser-UV for inactivation of virus in blood products. Blood 70(2):589–592, 1987

16. Puliafito CA, Stern D, Krueger RR, et al: High-speed photography of excimer laser ablation of the cornea. Arch Ophthalmol 105(99):1255–1259, 1987

17. Puliafito CA, Wong K, Steinert RF: Quantitative and ultrastructural studies of excimer laser ablation of the cornea at 193 and 248 nanometers. Lasers Surg Med 7(2):155–159, 1987

18. Schroder E, Dardenne MU, Neuhann T, et al: An ophthalmic excimer laser for corneal surgery. Am J Ophthalmol 102:472–473, 1987

19. Sutcliffe E, Srinivasan R: Dynamics of UV laser ablation of organic polymer surfaces. J Applied Phys 60:3313, 1986

20. Taylor RS, Singleton DL, Pareskevopoulous G: Effect of optical pulse duration on xenon chloride ablation of polymers and biologic tissues. Appl Phys Lett 50(25), June 22, 1987

21. Troutman RC, Veronneau-Troutman S, Jakobiec FA, et al: A new laser for collagen wounding in corneal and strabismus surgery: A preliminary report. Trans Am Ophthalmol Soc 84:117–132, 1986

22. Trentacoste J, Thompson K, Parrish RK 2nd, et al: Mutagenic potential of 193-nm excimer laser on fibroblasts in tissue culture. Ophthalmology 92(2):125–129, 1987

Index

Note: Page numbers in italics *indicate illustrations;
those followed by t indicate tables.*

ISBN 0-397-50962-6